Against Relativism

AGAINST RELATIVISM

*Cultural Diversity
and the Search for
Ethical Universals
in Medicine*

RUTH MACKLIN

New York   Oxford
OXFORD UNIVERSITY PRESS
1999

Oxford University Press

Oxford   New York
Athens   Auckland   Bangkok   Bogotá   Buenos Aires   Calcutta
Cape Town   Chennai   Dar es Salaam   Delhi   Florence   Hong Kong   Istanbul
Karachi   Kuala Lumpur   Madrid   Melbourne   Mexico City   Mumbai
Nairobi   Paris   São Paulo   Singapore   Taipei   Tokyo   Toronto   Warsaw

and associated companies in
Berlin   Ibadan

Copyright © 1999 by Oxford University Press, Inc.

Published by Oxford University Press, Inc.
198 Madison Avenue, New York, New York 10016

Oxford is a registered trademark of Oxford University Press

Library of Congress Cataloging-in-Publication Data
Macklin, Ruth, 1938–
Against relativism :
cultural diversity and the search for ethical universals in medicine /
Ruth Macklin.
p.   cm.
Includes bibliographical references and index.
ISBN 0-19-511632-1
1. Medical ethics — Cross-cultural studies.
2. Transcultural medical care — Moral and ethical aspects.
3. Ethical absolutism.   4. Ethical relativism.
5. Cultural relativism.
I. Title.
R725.5 .M33   1999
174'.2 — ddc21   98-44063

1 3 5 7 9 8 6 4 2

Printed in the United States of America
on acid-free paper

Preface

In 1992 I was awarded a grant by the Ford Foundation to conduct research and to serve as a consultant to the Foundation's program officers, their grantees, and others in developing countries throughout the world. The focus of the projects was ethics and reproductive health and sexuality. In my initial grant proposal to the Ford Foundation, I promised to address questions related to cultural relativity and ethical relativism. In that proposal I wrote: "A long-standing debate in ethics and public policy focuses on the fact that ethical beliefs and practices may vary from one place to another, giving rise to the question whether there are any overarching or universal ethical precepts. It remains true that cultural beliefs and practices in some parts of the world depart from the tenets that have come to embody respect for human rights in a large part of the modern world." The project sought to combine empirical information about actual customs and cultural practices gained in the course of my research with an analysis based on ethical theory and widely accepted principles of biomedical ethics. This book takes the inquiry beyond the focus on reproductive health and sexuality into other topics in medicine and health care.

The first three chapters explore an array of general topics central to debates among philosophers and anthropologists surrounding cultural relativity and ethical relativism. While recounting the leading positions put forth by several philosophers, I make no attempt to settle the deep theoretical questions that lie at the foundations of ethics: What is the ultimate source of ethical universals? If universal ethical principles exist, how can conflicts between or among them be resolved? Can satisfactory ethics be built on a plurality of theoretical perspectives?

Chapters 4 through 8 address specific topics in bioethics through the lens of cultural diversity: the physician-patient relationship, disclosing a diagnosis of fatal illness, informed consent, brain death and organ transplantation, rituals surrounding birth and death, female genital mutilation, sex selection of offspring, fertility regulation, and biomedical research involving human subjects. The unsurprising conclusion of these various inquiries is that, while ethical relativism can be sustained for some cultural practices and traditions, for others it should be rejected as a pernicious doctrine. Actions or policies based on ethical relativism rooted in cultural diversity can have dire consequences for the health, well being, and the very lives of human beings.

One consequence of belief in an extreme version of ethical relativism is its inconsistency with the notion that fundamental human rights exist. Chapter 9 discusses various positions pertaining to human rights, along with the disagreement between those who endorse civil-political rights as human rights and those who support social-economic rights as human rights. I make no attempt to provide a solution to this decades-old debate, but try instead to locate those rights related to medicine and health that deserve to be considered human rights. The final chapter presents my conclusions, elucidating the concept of moral progress along the way. Ethical universals exist, but they should not be confused with moral absolutes. The existence of ethical universals is compatible with a variety of culturally relative interpretations. Such statements are mere assertions unless accompanied by lots of illustrative examples and cogent arguments. That is what I have sought to provide in this volume.

Ford Foundation program officers arranged meetings with individuals and groups in the regions I visited. The people with whom I met included physicians, lawyers, social scientists, academic researchers, clergy, personnel in Ministries of Health, other government employees, women's health advocates, representatives of numerous and varied nongovernmental organizations, journalists, and other philosophers and ethicists. Most of these activities were without incident and I was greeted with good will and collegiality in virtually all of my experiences.

It therefore came as a shock when I was viciously attacked by a group of faculty and students at Wellesley College following an invited lecture I delivered on "son preference" in India and East Asia. Members of the audience contended that I had no right, based on my single visit to that country, to talk about customs in India. One aggressive faculty member demanded to know whom I spoke with there and criticized me for not specifying my sources for all the statements I made in my lecture (the paper had about thirty footnotes, which I refrained from reading aloud). The one person from India whom I did identify by name was dismissed as "not credible" by the faculty member. One student asked what my motives were in going to India and in conducting this project.

Reeling with surprise from this attack, I asked the audience whether it would have been better if I had just discussed the ethical issues surrounding son preference in the abstract, without any reference to facts or circumstances in particular countries — India or anywhere else. To my surprise, an anthropologist and another faculty member in women's studies shouted "Yes!" in reply. I found this curious, if not dismaying. Philosophers are often criticized for being "abstract," "ahistorical," and "acontextual." My experience in applied ethics has overwhelmingly demonstrated that participants at conferences demand examples and a contextual background for ethical analyses. Here, in my effort to be contextual and concrete, I was vilified for my presumptuousness in talking about a culture in which I had not lived and which I had no credentials to study.

A dinner that evening included most of the faculty members who had been aggressive and outspoken in the attack following my lecture. The assault continued, but took on a new dimension. The two most critical faculty members referred to the text of my lecture as racist in tone and reflecting a colonialist mentality. I was accused of sounding like the "racist and colonialist" John Stuart Mill, admittedly one of my philosophical heroes (and a staunch feminist, to boot).

What was this all about, I wondered? When I asked for examples, they could provide none without the written text but said that I had used "coded" language. Still puzzled, I surmised that there must be an academic industry out there that has invented the code and is looking around for unsuspecting, naive people like me who unwittingly use code words that betray racist and colonialist attitudes. Perhaps there is a codebook that contains a glossary of such terms and these feminists and social scientists are among the cognoscenti. Readers interested in the content of my lecture that prompted this response can find the text in this book. It is the section on son preference that appears in Chapter 6, "Birth and Death."

But I am not entirely in the dark about the use of terminology that marks one as a racist or colonialist. After my visit to India I wrote an article on son preference and sex determination that was published in an Indian medical ethics journal. In the article I referred (in descriptive terms, I thought) to India and China as "traditional, male-dominated societies." A critical article written in reply described these words as "Macklin's value-loaded (rather colonial and racist) remarks." The view that people who are not from a particular culture may not even seek to describe that culture, much less criticize it, appears to be held in some circles. I discuss this view briefly in Chapter 7.

I have nevertheless taken the risk of using "coded" language throughout this book. Various chapters mention "Western" countries, "European and North American values," "reproductive rights," and women living in "oppressive cultures." In the eyes of some, simply using these terms marks one as a colonialist or neocolonialist. Chapter 3 recounts the same charge leveled by an Egyptian anthropologist against an American medical student who dared to write about female genital mutilation in Egypt and who innocently used the word "Western." Another feminist anthropologist is quoted in the same chapter as saying that universalistic pronouncements like "Female circumcision violates women's human rights" are "unfortunate."

What I think is going on in identifying certain language as "racist" and "colonialist" is the unspoken premise that people from one culture are not qualified to discuss the beliefs, attitudes, and behavior of people from another culture. Americans may not discuss women in India, men may not discuss problems of women, white people may not write about black people. Those who adhere to this view share some sort of code that they use to identify violators who deign to write about the "other." Invariably, our language will betray us as "racist" or "colonialist" because we are, in fact, outsiders. Merely trying to describe a situation, based on interviews, books, and articles invites criticism: "One can't arrogantly dismiss Macklin's narrative of the depressing lives of Indian women as a gutter inspector's job because she discusses a crucial subject. However, her one-sided projection

of Indian women as victims of Hindu religious traditions, dowry harass-
ment, and societal pressure to produce sons may generate paralysis which
we cannot afford. . . ."*

Attacks on this book are, therefore, likely to be forthcoming from at
least three prominent and probably overlapping sources. The first is postmodern academics who inhabit ivory towers and speak to one another in
the pages of their journals. They will no doubt object to my attempt to
simply describe the cultural practices and values I have observed or read
about in countries other than the United States. According to postmodern
dogma, objectivity does not exist anywhere in the world, and there is
surely no basis for universality in ethics. All values are derived from particular cultural or contextual experiences. Adherence to the doctrine of
ethical relativism is an unavoidable consequence of adherence to the dictates of postmodernism. In presenting arguments against relativism, this
book also rejects the postmodern thesis.

A second, related source of criticism is based on feminist standpoint
theory.† According to this view, self-consciousness about the inevitable
nearsightedness of one's standpoint is required, since all people are unselfconscious products of the environment in which they grow up. No one
can escape the influence of social location on theory or practice.‡ An outsider to a culture has no capacity, no authority, and therefore no right to
say anything about what goes on there.

A third likely source of attack comes from native inhabitants of the
country, culture, or region under discussion. Again, it is argued that for-
eigners lack intimate familiarity and long-standing acquaintance with the
culture they seek to describe, and therefore they have little capacity for ac-
curacy or in-depth understanding (except, perhaps, if the outsider happens
to be a trained anthropologist and goes there to live for years.). One example is the Egyptian woman anthropologist quoted in Chapter 6, who also

---

*Vibhuti Patel, "The Ethics of Gender Justice," *Medical Ethics*, Vol. 3, No. 4 (1995),
p. 65.

†I lack extensive acquaintance with the considerable literature in feminist theory, and
owe this brief description to a pre-publication reviewer of my manuscript.

‡Karen Lebacqz, "Feminism," (ed.) Warren T. Reich, *Encyclopedia of Bioethics*, 2nd
edition (New York: Macmillan, 1995), p. 810.

evinces feminist standpoint theory, in her vicious attack on an American male physician who depicted female genital mutilation as a terrible public health problem in Egypt.

Some shortcomings in the methodology of this book will be evident to readers. One shortcoming is the minimal amount of empirical data derived from reputable, published studies. Much of the information is drawn from interviews, meetings, and informal conversations. Although I believe that most of my sources were reliable, anecdotes and personal accounts are no substitute for carefully designed studies by social scientists. In places that make broad claims for cultures or countries, I plead guilty to drawing conclusions that appear to simplify an admittedly complex situation. At the same time, however, the effort throughout this book is to anchor philosophical arguments against relativism in the reality of living cultures and the people who inhabit them.

Bronx, N.Y.   R.M.
September 1998

Acknowledgments

I am grateful to the Ford Foundation for its support of two successive international projects on ethics and reproductive health. Much of the information in this book was gathered in the course of my visits to countries in Asia, Africa, and Latin America under those projects. Special thanks go to José Barzelatto, then the Director of the Ford Foundation's program in Reproductive Health, to Marjorie Muecke and Margaret Hempel, program officers in the Foundation's New York office, and to the Foundation's regional program officers who facilitated my interviews and meetings.

Some material in this book is adapted or excerpted from previously published articles. Small sections of Chapters 1 and 2 are taken from my chapter, "Universality of the Nuremburg Code," in George J. Annas and Michael A. Grodin (eds.), *The Nazi Doctors and the Nuremburg Code: Human Rights in Human Experimentation* (New York: Oxford University Press, 1992). Much of Chapter 5 was published as "Ethical Relativism in a Multicultural Society," in the *Kennedy Institute of Ethics Journal*, Vol. 8 (1998), and a short section of Chapter 7 is taken from my commentary, "Combatting the Potential for Abuse," in *Reproductive Health Matters*, Number 4 (1994), pp. 110–112. Some portions of Chapter 6 appeared in my chapter, "Justice in International Research," in Jeffrey Kahn, Anna Mastroianni, and Jeremy Sugarman (eds.), *Beyond Consent* (New York: Oxford University Press, 1998), and other portions in "International Research: Ethical Imperialism or Ethical Pluralism?" in *Accountability in Research* (1999). Parts of Chapter 1 and Chapter 10 are revised excerpts from "Moral Progress," which appeared in *Ethics*, published by the University of Chicago Press (copyright 1977 by The University of Chicago. All rights reserved). A few scattered paragraphs from various chapters were excerpted in an article entitled "A Defense of Fundamental Principles and Human Rights: A Response to Baker," in the *Kennedy Institute of Ethics Journal*, Vol. 8 (1998). I thank the editors and publishers for permission to use the material.

The encouragement of Jeffrey W. House at Oxford University Press was a great asset from beginning to end. A reviewer of the manuscript whose identity remains unknown to me made many helpful suggestions, almost all of which I used in making final revisions. Special thanks go to my friend, Dr. Marie Burnett, for her thorough editorial work on the entire manuscript and for her intellectual insights and moral support. Finally, I am grateful to all my international colleagues—those whom I met in the course of my Ford Foundation work and the many others with whom I continue to have ongoing discussions about the topics of this book.

Contents

Against Relativism

1

Cultural and Ethical Relativism

A long-standing debate surrounds the question whether ethics are relative to time and place. One side argues that there is no obvious source of a universal morality and that ethical rightness and wrongness are products of their cultural and historical setting. Opponents claim that even if a universal set of ethical norms has not yet been articulated or agreed upon, ethical relativism is a pernicious doctrine that must be rejected. The first group replies that the search for universal ethical precepts is a quest for the Holy Grail. The second group responds with the telling charge: If ethics were relative to time, place, and culture, then what the Nazis did was "right" for them, and there is no basis for moral criticism by anyone outside the Nazi society.

Both sides of this unsophisticated version of the debate appear to capture a kernel of truth. There is no denying that different cultures and historical eras exhibit a variety of moral beliefs and practices. The empirical facts revealed by anthropological research yield the descriptive thesis known as *cultural relativity*. But even if we grant that cultural relativity is an accurate description of the world's diversity, whether anything follows for normative ethics is an entirely different question. Do the facts of cultural relativity compel the conclusion that what is right or wrong can be determined only by the beliefs and practices within a particular culture or subculture? Does it mean that there can be no overarching ethical principles that could be used to assess the rightness or wrongness of actions or practices in different places or at different times?

Confusions about ethical relativism abound. I was reminded of this after I had finished delivering an introduction to a conference at the Holocaust Memorial Museum on the behavior of physicians in Nazi Germany. My remarks included the comment that ethical judgments are complex affairs and have many determinants. I went on to say that people often have strong moral sentiments that underlie or motivate ethical judgments even when they try to provide rational, objective justifications for their ethical conclusions. The strength of a person's moral sentiment on a particular topic colors the objectivity of the ethical judgment, leading that person to see an issue differently from others who stand at a distance from the situation and whose assessments are more objective. My point was that survivors of the Holocaust and people who lost entire families at the hands of the Nazis would naturally experience deeper emotions than people who had not undergone those experiences, and the two groups might therefore come to different conclusions about contemporary issues like the ethics of assisted suicide, voluntary euthanasia, genetic interventions, and human experimentation.

When I had finished speaking, another participant, a historian who specializes in Holocaust studies, came up to me and said, "I see you're an absolutist." "No," I replied, "I'm not." Without further explanation, I added, "I'm certainly not an absolutist. I don't believe that exceptionless ethical rules exist." The historian then said, "But you seemed to be rejecting relativism." "Oh yes, I replied, that's certainly true. I reject ethical relativism as firmly as I reject absolutism." We did not have the opportunity to pursue the conversation. Later on, I was as amazed at the historian's own statements in the course of her contributions to a panel discussion as she was at mine. She asserted at one point that "Context is everything" and at another juncture that "Relativism is, of course, the only reasonable position."

Clearly, we need a richer vocabulary than this simple exchange employed. It is a common belief that "absolutism" is the opposite of "relativism"; anyone who rejects ethical relativism must be an ethical absolutist. That view is quite mistaken. My response to the historian implied as much, but I did not have the chance to explain. What amazed me about the historian's remarks was that she made them not at a conference of anthropologists discussing the practices of indigenous peoples who have remained isolated from mainstream culture, but at a symposium about the behavior of German doctors in the Holocaust. If there is any time and place in which unqualified ethical judgments appear sound and uncontroversial, it is the era of Nazi Germany that witnessed the genocide of more than six million "undesirables," the unspeakable horrors of the concentration camps, and the atrocities committed by German doctors in the name of medical science. Yet so pervasive is the dogma of postmodernism that everything is "socially constructed" that it can lead an otherwise sober historian (who was most certainly not a Holocaust denier or a Nazi sympathizer) to contend that "context is everything."

Consider the following practices: female genital mutilation; requirement of husbands' permission for their wives to participate in research; self-immolation of widows in India. Female genital mutilation (politely but misleadingly termed "female circumcision" or "surgery") is a ritual practiced in some African countries. Its defenders dismiss Western condemnation as a misplaced failure to show respect for African traditions. Spousal authorization for medical procedures is a commonly accepted custom in many developing countries, and its defenders contend that the custom embodies the traditional marital roles of husband and wife. Self-immolation of widows in India is also defended by an appeal to the significance of the marital bond in Hindu religion and morality (however, there is no corresponding tradition of self-immolation of widowers). In addition, apologists contend that it is a genuinely voluntary act on the part of a newly widowed woman.[1] A defender of any of these customs can point to cultural significance, tradition, or religion. But even if such customs can be distinguished from raw exercise of power or exploitation by the strong over the weak, why should the defense that they are religious or cultural traditions render them immune from moral criticism by outsiders to the culture?

The concept of "culture" itself is ambiguous and often means different things to different people. One critic of the sloppy use of the term writes that "most of the time, *culture* is a lazy, trendy substitute for a more specific word." The anthropological use of the term "refers to the total way of life of a discrete society, its traditions, habits, beliefs, and art. . . ."[2] A culture, in this purportedly "genuine" sense, is defined by certain constant features that differentiate it from other cultures in other times or places. The anthropologist Margaret Mead took "culture" to mean "the systematic body of learned behavior which is transmitted from parents to children."[3] The anthropological linguist, Edward Sapir, contended that a genuine culture is not an externally imposed set of rules or forms or a "passively accepted heritage from the past," but rather a "way of life" inseparably linked to the beliefs, desires, and interests of its members.[4] When I refer in these chapters to "genuine cultures" or "cultural tradition in its true sense," I adopt the general meaning defined by these scholars.

People make cross-cultural ethical judgments all the time. Westerners criticize authoritarian nations that prohibit political dissent and imprison political opponents. International moral outrage followed the reports of ethnic cleansing in Bosnia and the rape of Muslim women by soldiers as a deliberate weapon of war during that bloody conflict. Women and men throughout the world contend that female circumcision both harms and wrongs the girls and women who are subjected to it, and even defenders of women's right to abortion affirm their opposition to forced abortions that have occurred in China. Although defenders of each of these practices can be found within the culture or country where the conduct occurs, there is something about these actions that prompts almost universal condemnation. The justifications that underlie these ethical judgments rely on fundamental principles that I maintain can be universally applied. And those principles are the underpinnings of at least some of what are recognized today as human rights.

It is sometimes hard to tell whether a rejection of cross-cultural judgments stems from a postmodern challenge to ethical universality or from a concern for politically oppressed minorities. There is often a tendency to defend the actions of marginalized groups even if those same actions would be condemned if carried out by the dominant or more powerful group. I participated in a meeting in Chile in which a young woman told a story that shocked my Western (or "Northern," to use the currently preferred term) ethical sensibilities. The majority of Chileans are of European origin, but there remain a few scattered indigenous groups outside the large cities. One such group continues to practice a traditional ritual in which newborn infants are sacrificed. The government of Chile forbade this practice by law and succeeded in bringing it to a halt. But when the region where the indigenous group dwelt experienced a severe drought, causing suffering and hardship to the people, they contended that the gods were punishing them for their failure to carry on the ritual sacrifices required by their religion and blamed the state for its prohibition of human sacrifice.

The woman who recounted this story defended the stance of this ethnic group and condemned the government for imposing its power and authority on the weaker indigenous group. I countered by saying that the group was doing something ethically unacceptable in killing babies and, further, that there was no scientific validity to their belief that human sac-

rifice could prevent drought or that to resume the sacrifice would end the
drought. In reply, the woman who had told the story scorned my ethical
concerns and considered me an unenlightened victim of narrow Western
(Northern) scientific and ethical dogmatism. "That is their belief; the belief in modern science is your belief. Both are simply beliefs." Scientific
notions of causality have no more validity than ethical judgments. Both
are up for grabs. This position illustrates a form of "epistemological" relativism, distinct from yet related to ethical relativism. Epistemological relativism is the view that systems of belief about the natural world differ from
one culture to another and so, too, do the ways of justifying beliefs about
"matters of fact." No one belief system can be held to be more valid than
the next. Beliefs based on modern science are no more true than beliefs
based on myth or superstition.

     Although it is indisputable that different nations, cultures, and reli-
gious and ethnic groups adhere to different norms of behavior, it is possible to analyze individual conduct and social practices by seeing how they
conform to fundamental ethical principles. Whether those principles are
universal, applicable to all societies at all times in history, is a matter of ongoing debate. Whether general ethical principles are so vague and indeter-
minate as to be useless is another point of contention. It is certainly the
case that general principles are open to a variety of particular interpretations, and these have evolved over time.

     Consider, for example, one of the leading principles in bioethics, "re-
spect for persons."[5] This general principle is open to interpretations that
depart from the most common Western version that focuses on individual
autonomy. Even the idea that there is a single "Western" concept of autonomy has been challenged. A Spanish scholar has argued that the term
autonomy acquired different meanings in the United States and in
Europe. In the ethical literature in the United States, this scholar
contends, autonomy is defined as the capacity to act intentionally, with
understanding, and without controlling influences. This is an "empirical"
concept of autonomy. On the other hand, European ethicists often interpret the principle of autonomy as a "transcendental" term derived from
the writings of the philosopher Immanuel Kant: "the capacity of human
reason to impose absolute moral laws upon itself." These two meanings are

so disparate that an autonomous person according to the European point of view may not act autonomously from the American perspective because of constraints such as ignorance or coercion.[6]

These contrasting conceptions of autonomy are probably of greater interest to philosophers than to physicians who earnestly strive to respect their patients' autonomy, but they demonstrate the subtleties involved in taking account of transcultural interpretations of ethical concepts. In seeking a bridge between these conceptions, I define *autonomy* as "the human capacity for self-rule or self-determination." Following from this definition is the moral principle that *the autonomy of persons ought to be respected.*[7]

This, in turn, poses the further challenge of understanding the concept of a "person," a task that has occupied philosophers throughout the ages. While I recognize that certain metaphysical assumptions underlie the position I develop, I have chosen to avoid a digression into metaphysics in this book. Nevertheless, it is critically important to distinguish between the claim that the concept of a "person" does not have a single, unequivocal meaning (which may be true even within a single culture) and the quite different claim that the *value* accorded the individual person varies from one society or culture to another. It is undeniable that some societies place the interests of the community or group over the interests of the individual person, whereas it is often noted that the United States is a country in which the individual "reigns supreme." When the interests of the larger group ought to take precedence over those of the individual is an important question of normative ethics, and the answer may vary from one place to another. But it would be an uncritical concession to ethical relativism to say that whatever value a particular society accords to individuals is therefore morally right.

The contrast between the Western world and the East is frequently noted in this connection. A Chinese colleague mentioned that "respect for persons" has a long history in China and is part of the Confucian heritage. He acknowledged, however, that the traditional Chinese interpretation of the "respect for persons" principle did not include autonomy.[8] It is also unlikely that the principle in China has traditionally been understood to include *equal* respect for persons, which would grant full status to women. Analogously, Islamic scholars contend that the Koran contains many points of Islamic law that require respect for women as persons, but that respect does not extend to granting women decision-making autonomy. Historically, of course, the interpretation that mandates equal respect for women has not prevailed in the West either. This poses the related question of historical ethical relativism: Is ethics relative to the historical time in which actions and practices that are today considered unethical were widely practiced and considered to be right?[9]

Some cultural differences are so substantial that they seem to defy comparison. At an informal meeting of program officers working in Nigeria for a major American philanthropic foundation, I had the task of describing the international project I was engaged in and explaining how the field of bioethics might help to address the problems the project dealt with.[10] None of the program officers was a native Nigerian, although not all were Americans. As a sometime user and defender of the well-known principles of bioethics, I stated and explicated the principles of nonmaleficence, beneficence, respect for persons, and prominent principles of justice.[11] When I had finished, one participant asked: "Are these the only fundamental ethical principles?" This penetrating question posed a major challenge.

These were highly educated people who were unacquainted with the field of bioethics. They wanted to know whether other ethical principles could be put on a par with the ones now so familiar (but also challenged) in bioethics. Turning the challenge back to them, I asked if they could provide examples of candidates for coequal principles. One person proposed "respect for tradition." Never having heard this proposed as an ethical principle, I wondered whether it should qualify as one. If it does, is it on a par as a fundamental principle with "respect for persons" or the ethical imperative to strive to bring about more benefits than harms? "Maintain respect for tradition" is a customary norm within many societies and operates as a conservative force for maintaining the status quo. It also functions as a practical and possibly also a moral maxim for anthropologists conducting fieldwork.

The motive that lay behind the participant's suggestion of "respect for tradition" as an ethical principle was her observation that it can conflict with one or more of the three principles I had elucidated in my presentation. Moreover, working with various ethnic and religious groups in Nigeria, she often encountered "respect for tradition" being used as a justification for practices that diverge from Western customs and conflict with Western ethical standards of conduct. Two leading examples are the ritual of female genital mutilation and early marriage of girls as young as 9 or 10 years old. Seeking to avoid the evident problems arising from treating "respect for tradition" as a fundamental ethical principle, another participant at that meeting in Nigeria objected to the proposed candidate with the remark: "We try not to use the word *tradition;* we only speak of *history.*"

Another discussion, at a different meeting in Nigeria, this time a workshop consisting of Nigerian medical professionals, social scientists, and grassroots health advocates, attempted to get an answer to the question, "How acceptable is abortion in Nigerian society?" One participant said that in becoming modern, it is important not to destroy the traditions of society. Another referred to "the traditional culture." Seeking to get beyond the standard replies that appeal to "traditions" and "culture," one woman insisted that the word *culture* is used to cover up lots of things. Men define "culture" as it suits their needs and values, she said. This led to a discussion of the meaning of these terms and the purposes served when people appeal to "respect for tradition" to defend their particular ethical point of view. Women's health advocates argued that it is necessary to be cautious in using the words *traditional* and *cultural* when discussing customs and practices that are harmful to women. One person said that many practices in Africa today are not "traditional" in the sense that they arise from African roots. Rather, they are the product of contact with the West and the heritage of colonialism. Women have been pushed out of positions they traditionally held prior to colonial power. When it comes to abortion, every culture and society throughout history has included traditional healers who sought to help women end their unwanted pregnancies.

Within cultures as well as across cultures, some ethical values have greater importance than others. Some ethical matters deal with basic ways human beings treat each other, whereas others shade into what is more like etiquette. The recognition of different levels of ethical significance enables a case to be made for a modified form of ethical relativism. To reject an ethically unacceptable brand of relativism—the extreme version—does not require us to accept the view that no ethical values whatsoever can be relative to a culture or region. An example of this middle ground between ethical universalism and ethical relativism is the difference in how privacy and confidentiality are viewed in China and elsewhere in Asia in contrast to in the West.

In daily life the traditional Chinese culture has not recognized or respected either informational privacy or physical privacy. A rather trivial yet amusing example, recounted by a North American woman who was living in China, was an experience she had in the workplace.[12] As in many countries, people often bring their lunch to work. My colleague was surprised to find her coworkers opening up each others' lunch bags (including her own) to find out their contents. In the United States, the contents of a lunch bag are normally not viewed as something intimate or intrinsically private. When lunchtime rolls around, coworkers sit at a table and display for all to see what they have brought for lunch. But it would surely violate a cultural norm for someone in this country to peer into the lunchbag of another without asking permission. Would it be an ethical transgression? It would surely be less of an invasion of privacy than reading another person's diary or looking through the contents of someone's desk drawers. But in our culture, to peer into a coworker's lunchbag without permission would be a transgression of someone's personal property and therefore, an invasion of privacy. We value informational privacy and spatial privacy, and place a high value on personal property. In the West, we elevate the protection of these forms of privacy to a "right"; but surely a glimpse into a coworker's lunchbag is not a violation of a basic right. It involves a social norm—something a bit more serious than mere etiquette, yet surely not approaching the level of a violation of a universal ethical principle.

Although respect for privacy is much more a Western value, even in China and other Eastern cultures some respect for boundaries is an accepted norm. A Chinese colleague recounted this next example during a visit I made to China. Patients who were unclothed or partially clothed were subjected to a medical examination in full view of a group of visitors to the hospital. Despite their manifest discomfort, they submitted to this indignity without complaint because their physicians told them that visitors were to observe the medical exams. Physicians in China are so revered and respected that patients almost always comply with their orders. But the discomfort of the patients demonstrated that bodily privacy is a boundary that would not be overstepped even in China were it not for the authority commanded by the physician.

However, embarrassment over intrusions of bodily privacy might not extend to other realms. In the early 1970s an American colleague visited China to study the health care delivery system there. When he saw the names of patients, along with their diagnoses, displayed in a public place, he inquired through his interpreter whether the people did not consider this an invasion of their privacy. The interpreter replied that he could not properly translate the question because there was no word for privacy in Mandarin Chinese. If the language lacks a word for privacy, it is a foregone conclusion that ethical prohibitions relating to privacy will be similarly lacking. Yet it does not follow that there is no way of describing and ultimately condemning the Chinese doctor's action of ordering his patients to undergo medical examinations in front of strangers. Perhaps the Confucian version of the principle "respect for persons" could justify moral condemnation of the physician's behavior. It is the Western version of the same principle that provides a basis for making ethical judgments relating to privacy in our own culture.

When it comes to lack of informational privacy, disclosure of details about people's personal lives has a long tradition in China. Historically, everything was told to the patriarch. People took their troubles and voluntarily reported private events in their lives to the patriarch. People accepted this practice and presumably felt no sense of intrusion into their privacy. Sometimes the patriarch revealed such information to others, and other times not. After 1949, the head of the work unit came to serve as a functional replacement for the traditional patriarch. In recent times it has become the head of the work unit to whom things are routinely told. A Chinese philosopher described this situation as very different from an employer–employee relationship in the West.[13] He said it is more analogous to the patriarch's role in the old regime. But with recent changes, especially the opening of China to a free-market economy, the situation in the workplace is now becoming more like the Western employer–employee relationship. This is a telling example of how political and economic changes create a need for a revision of traditional values in order to adapt to the new circumstances.

Cultural relativity is apparent in other situations concerning informational privacy. Breaches of confidentiality that would be viewed as wrong in the West are taken for granted and widely accepted in China. One example is the public postings of women's menstrual cycles, not only in the hospital or clinic but also in the workplace. The factory or work unit is frequently the site of various forms of health care monitoring and delivery. This arrangement accounts, in part, for the well-developed health infrastructure in China. In this typical circumstance, disclosure of personal or intimate information about health status is expected and does not, as a rule, have harmful consequences to the individual whose data are made public. According to Western values, however, individuals would be wronged, even if they are not harmed, in these situations of disclosure of personal health-related information.

Nevertheless, in China as in the West, some breaches of confidentiality could harm the individual and would then be regarded as wrong. An example that came out in a meeting with researchers on human sexuality and AIDS was that of disclosure to the work unit leader that a worker was HIV positive. This resulted in the worker's dismissal from his job and possible inability to obtain another job. Even though the Chinese government and employers defend the requirement that physicians report to employers any individuals tested for HIV and found to be positive, the breach of confidentiality is considered ethically unacceptable by the Chinese academics with whom I spoke because of the social and economic harm it typically produces for the affected individuals and possibly also their families.

In a culture like China's, where there is no recognized right to privacy or confidentiality, to invade an individual's privacy or to breach confidentiality would not automatically be viewed as wrong. This is partly because of norms that have prevailed for centuries, reflecting the different status of the individual in Western and Eastern cultures. Even in our Western philosophical tradition, privacy seems to be a middle-level concept rather than a fundamental ethical value like liberty. Privacy does appear to be a culturally relative value, one that can vary from one culture to the next without violating a fundamental ethical principle. However, when the invasion of privacy or breach of confidentiality causes demonstrable physical, psychological, or social harm to the individual, as in the examples given earlier, then it can be judged ethically wrong because of these harms and not because it is a violation of a fundamental right to privacy.

The concept of privacy plays a rather special role in the context of Constitutional protections, as interpreted by the United States Supreme Court, as I learned from an experience with a group in Mexico that is working toward decriminalization of the abortion laws there.[14] This group, which goes by the Spanish acronym GIRE (El Grupo de Información en Reproducción Elegida) had prepared a memorandum in advance of our meeting, which was to focus on strategies that might work in Mexico to reform their abortion laws. The memorandum began by referring to "the differences between the set of beliefs and values our countries are founded upon." More specifically, the memo stated "the fact that in the U.S. the individual is the focus around which social organization revolves, whereas in Mexico, society takes that place." This supposition was provided as background to the specific question we were to address concerning abortion: "Can we, in Mexico, propose abortion as a right within the realm of a right to privacy?" I responded by agreeing that the value placed on the individual is probably stronger in the United States than anywhere else in the world. However, I questioned whether Mexico is as far from the United States in that respect as the question in the document presupposed.

First of all, in Mexico there does not exist the skepticism and rejection of the concept of human rights or individual rights that can be found in China and some African countries. Although it is true that some people in Mexico (especially those representing traditional Roman Catholic religious views) deny the concept of reproductive rights, their rejection is limited to the "reproductive" aspect and not to the fundamental concept of rights. However, a provision of the Mexican Constitution explicitly mentions a general reproductive right: Article 4 asserts the right of each individual or couple to decide responsibly on the number and spacing of their children. This, along with ample evidence that Mexicans in every socioeconomic class express their social and political concerns in the language of rights, led me to question whether the fundamental value system in Mexico is as different as the GIRE memo appeared to suggest. It is certainly reasonable to ask whether the value of privacy is the correct one for Mexicans seeking abortion reform to use as a basis for women's right to choice regarding abortion, contraceptives, or sterilization. That is a question about the proper justification for claims about reproductive rights and the best strategy to secure them. It is not the question as put to me by GIRE: whether the individual or the larger society is the focus around which social organization revolves. Once the concept of rights is introduced and acknowledged, the rights in question are, for the most part, understood as belonging to individuals, although it is true that rights are also claimed by indigenous groups or social classes that have been oppressed or marginalized.

A different question posed in the GIRE memo pertained to arguments that appeal to the value of privacy: "How do you handle the difference between those who support abortion on the premises of privacy and those who—even within the U.S. itself—would like to support it upon another footing, for example, upon a social agreement as opposed to a judicial determination?" To answer these questions it was necessary to explain the relationship between law and ethics, with particular reference to the U.S. judicial system.

I explained to the group that the concept of privacy entered into the general debates over abortion in the United States because of the 1973 Supreme Court decision in *Roe v. Wade*. When the court reviewed that case, it had to identify some Constitutional precedent for determining that women have a Constitutional right to seek abortions. The court's line of reasoning employed a case from 1965, *Griswold v. Connecticut*, which held that states could not outlaw a married woman's use of birth control. The Court's argument in the Griswold case rested on the notion that what married couples do "in the privacy of their bedroom" is not a matter for state regulation. In that ruling, the Court cited an unenumerated constitutional "right to privacy" implicit in the Bill of Rights and the Fourteenth Amendment. In *Roe*, however, the privacy relationship was that between doctor and patient (the wording in *Roe v. Wade* made the abortion decision a private matter between the woman and her doctor). Hence the importation of the concept of privacy to the abortion debate in the United States had a great deal to do with the Supreme Court's mode of argumentation and much less to do with privacy as a value that serves as a moral underpinning for abortion rights. In fact, the right to privacy has been controversial among lawyers and judges who are reluctant to recognize novel unenumerated rights.[15]

It is perhaps more significant that a subsequent U.S. Supreme Court decision that affirmed a woman's Constitutional right to abortion did not even mention privacy. *Casey v. Planned Parenthood Association of Southeastern Pennsylvania*,[16] decided in 1992, actually shifted the reasoning away from a privacy-based Constitutional right toward a liberty-based right. The Court interpreted the liberty clause of the Fourteenth Amendment in support of its reaffirmation of the constitutional right to abortion, drawing on past cases recognizing rights to bodily integrity and "a person's most basic decisions about family and parenthood." A basic right to terminate pregnancy was affirmed because it is a central aspect of the protected sphere of decision-making.[17]

The main point of my explanation to members of GIRE in Mexico was to note that the values that the Supreme Court uses as a basis for its arguments are ones that it has to find in the U.S. Constitution or in previous Supreme Court rulings. These may or may not be the same values one would use in a moral argument supporting a woman's right to abortion. I expressed my own view that liberty is a much more fundamental right than privacy in the United States and would be more applicable as a basis for abortion rights in the Mexican context. Societies that are less communitarian than the United States may recognize a strong sense of liberty against the dictates of the state, even while they place less value on individual privacy in the context of the community or family.

The question in GIRE's memorandum about basing abortion rights on "a social agreement as opposed to a judicial determination" also requires a distinction between ethical values and the governmental system that transforms such values into law. The reason abortion rights are supported by a judicial determination in the United States is that a Supreme Court ruling is the only way of ensuring that a particular right is guaran-

teed as a Constitutional right. Other rights may be granted by state legisla-
tures or by a federal law enacted by Congress. But a Constitutional right is
deeper, more fundamental, and the judicial determination of abortion
rights in the United States is a function of the role played by the tripartite
system of government and the different methods for establishing a legal
right. Once we leave the realm of constitutional rights, as specified in any
country's constitution or interpreted by a body like the Supreme Court, we
are in more contested territory. It is relatively easy to consult documents
and court cases to determine which legal rights have been enunciated, but
much harder to ascertain which rights are properly to be considered *human* rights. Despite their mention in numerous international declarations
and conventions, the meaning of *human rights* remains elusive and often
hotly contested.

       To determine whether cross-cultural judgments are sound requires
taking a step beyond the type of ethical analysis used for moral judgments
normally made within a cultural context. In the intracultural situation, we
begin with a description of the act or practice under scrutiny. The analysis
starts with a value-neutral description, insofar as that is possible. (Some
may argue that value-neutral descriptions are never possible, but I think
that view is mistaken.) The analysis proceeds by identifying relevant facts
and background circumstances, including an account of why this information is morally relevant. What counts as a justification will depend on
which ethical theory, principles, perspective, or approach one takes when
conducting an ethical analysis. Adherents of ethical principles employ
one or more of the well-known quartet in bioethics; a rights theorist looks
to see which, if any, rights have been violated; a casuist presumably begins without principles or theories, but those elements often lurk in the
background and come to the fore at the point of final justification. Feminists use one of the approaches that have come to be associated with the
various versions of feminist ethics: examining power relations between
men and women and oppression of women, making the notion of "caring"
central to the analysis or emphasizing "gender awareness" and "gender
sensitivity."

       What all these approaches have in common is the presumption that,
given a shared cultural background, ethical judgments are both meaning-

ful and valid. A moral nihilist rejects the possibility of ethical judgments altogether, as does the radical subjectivist. If the subjectivist's views can be characterized as "What's right for me is right for me, what's right for you is right for you," then criticisms of another's actions always lack validity or, worse, are altogether meaningless. There is no point to even talking about ethics. But if we begin with the assumption that making moral judgments of other people's actions is a legitimate enterprise, then the task is to justify such judgments by appealing to some shared values.

We have to start somewhere. If shared moral values do exist within cultures, what is the source of moral disagreement when that occurs? At least three obvious sources of disagreement are evident when controversies exist within a country or culture. The first lies in disagreement about facts or probabilities in the situation under analysis. Ethical debates that rely on assessments of the consequences of an action or policy typically illustrate this sort of disagreement. For example, opponents in recent debates concerning the acceptability of physician-assisted suicide dispute what would happen if physicians were legally permitted to help their patients to die. One side argues that physicians would be all too willing to save time and money caring for chronically ill patients and would write lethal prescriptions for vulnerable, elderly patients whose suffering could be relieved by more attention to palliative care. The other side envisions a different set of consequences, whereby only those patients suffering untreatable pain would be given the lethal prescriptions, and careful safeguards would prevent abuse.

The second type of disagreement surrounds the moral status of entities central to the case or situation. The abortion controversy is one case in point, where the moral status of embryonic or fetal life is disputed. Another example is that of anencephalic infants as a source of organs for transplantation. One side argues that anencephalic infants lack a brain and will inevitably die in a short while and therefore have a "lower" moral status that can permit taking their organs to save the lives of other infants. Opponents claim that the anencephalic is still a human infant and deserves the same respect as other living beings, from whom organs may not be removed until after death.

The third source of disagreement occurs when people place different priorities on values or principles that conflict in a particular situation. An example is the controversy about overriding Jehovah's Witnesses parents' refusal of a blood transfusion for their child and other cases in which parents refuse to consent to a treatment. One side argues that parents' rights over their minor children extend to refusal of medical treatments—even those deemed necessary to preserve life, while the other side places limits on parental decision-making. Both sides recognize parental rights of decision-making in general, but they disagree over whether the value of preserving a child's life or health may override that of respect for parental authority.

One or more of these sources of disagreement may be present in any ethical controversy. Sometimes an ethical resolution is possible in these different types of intracultural disagreement, and sometimes it is not. The contribution that a clear ethical analysis can make is to identify the source or sources of disagreement and thereby determine whether a resolution can be forthcoming. In cross-cultural ethical judgments, an additional step is necessary. That is the task of showing that ethical concepts or perspectives from outside the culture's accepted value framework are (or ought to be) relevant and applicable to the culture's traditions and practices. One way this could be done is to demonstrate that the culture already recognizes this particular ethical value in another sphere of activity but has so far neglected to apply that ethical concept to the practice under scrutiny, as the following example from our own history demonstrates.

The subsequent granting of rights to groups that were initially denied those rights illustrates the evolution of this moral concept. The Constitution and the Bill of Rights established the centrality of individual rights under the U.S. legal system. But amendments were needed before basic constitutional provisions, such as the right to liberty, were held to be applicable to black as well as to white Americans and the right to vote was applied to women and to former slaves as well as to white men. People from other cultures with a very different history contend that individualism is taken to an extreme in the United States and that this excessive individualism is unique to our culture. Critics from Asian and African countries claim that their cultures have legitimate values that depart from American individualism. Their lack of recognition of all of the rights embedded in

American society is not an ethical deficiency, they claim, but a cultural difference.

Of course it is hard, if not impossible, to escape one's own cultural biases. At the same time, changes take place within cultures when a visionary or courageous group seeks to alter the status quo. The women's movement in developing countries around the world today demonstrates how groups within a culture can come to recognize as injustice behavior that the majority in the culture takes for granted as "natural," inevitable, or part of its traditional heritage. Examples from two different countries are illustrative.

In the Philippines,[18] many people perceive diseases that afflict them as "natural" and, therefore, not subject to control. This perception exists on the part of people who use the services of traditional healers as well as the healers themselves. This is one manifestation of a tendency toward "fatalism" as a general cultural trait. Many Filipinos believe that "God will take care of things," an attitude reflected in the broader cultural phenomenon of lack of planning for the future. A fatalistic attitude or a resigned acceptance of the status quo extends to human affairs as well as to natural phenomena like the periodic eruptions of Mount Pinatubo, the volcano. People's perceptions of what is not subject to control or change also includes violence women experience at the hands of men. Battering of women is a serious and widespread problem. Yet because it has been a long-standing practice in Filipino culture, it is viewed as "natural." Interestingly, during the period surrounding the birth of a child women are granted special "concessions" by men. Uncharacteristically, men perform household chores during this period. Also during this period they refrain from beating their wives. However, these special concessions do not last beyond the postpartum period.

As in many other developing countries, women's health activists in the Philippines are seeking to change the traditional healers' view that violence against women is "natural" and that efforts to change this pattern would be futile. Women's health advocates also work at the grassroots level directly with women, trying to empower women within the family and the community. But first they must tackle the fundamental belief that underlies an acceptance of violence against women, the belief that such behavior is "natural" and therefore cannot be changed. If non-Filipinos were to propose attempts to change such beliefs and the violence that flows from them, the outsiders might be criticized for trying to impose alien beliefs and to change cultural traditions. That has been the response in Africa—including by some African women—to the concerns of Western feminists about female genital mutilation.

A popular stereotype holds that Mexican and other Latin cultures are traditionally *macho* in their attitude toward women. Accounts by women activists in Mexico depict the dominant value of *machismo* that creates in men a desire to prove their masculinity by having many children. Whether it is their wives or their mistresses who bear the children, credit goes to the men for fathering numerous offspring. A Mexican social anthropologist notes that the prevalent values of patriarchal Mexican culture make the roles of motherhood and fatherhood central elements in the gender construction of masculinity and femininity: "Until recent years, popular sayings included: 'To be a man is to be the father of more than four.'" A saying pertaining to women is considerably less charitable: "Women . . . were to be kept 'like shotguns, loaded and in the corner.' That is to say, pregnant and marginalized when it came to important matters."[19]

In both the Filipino and Mexican situations, dominant cultural beliefs and practices have perpetuated violence or other forms of coercion directed at women. If dominant cultural patterns deserve respect and continued adherence, as ethical relativism would appear to dictate, what can be the basis for an ethical critique of those practices? Must we conclude that violence against women is ethically permissible as an expression of dominant cultural values? A defender of "respect for tradition" might reply that these are not genuine examples of cultural traditions. Not every attitude or practice within a culture embodies a tradition in the way that religious and other rituals do. Violence against and domination of women in Mexico and the Philippines is a telling example of exploitation of the powerful over the less powerful, but it does not represent a *cultural* tradition in the true sense of the term. Violence against women exists in every culture, even in societies that profess gender equality and strive through laws and other reforms to achieve gender justice.

This reply is reasonable, but it relies on the intuitive ability to grasp the difference between treatment of women that embodies a genuine cultural tradition of distribution of gender roles, on the one hand, and the abuse by men of their greater power and authority, on the other. However, intuition is a notoriously poor guide to anything. Consider the following example from China, a country that retains a strong Confucian tradition despite the overlay of a half-century of Communist rule. This example demonstrates the power of the mother-in-law in an alliance with her son. At a meeting of Chinese reproductive health professionals and policymakers, a physician described the case as "an old example from years ago."

A woman in a village had three children, all girls. She did not want more children, but her husband and mother-in-law did not want her to be sterilized. They wanted her to continue having children. The ethical issue was presented as a dilemma for the physician: Should she sterilize the woman or follow the wishes of the patient's husband and mother-in-law? The physician tried to persuade the mother-in-law and husband to agree to the woman's sterilization, but that attempt failed.

What would be the consequences for the woman if the physician counseled her to go ahead with the sterilization? Everyone at the meeting concurred that the consequence would be that the husband would divorce her. Because the husband and mother-in-law wanted sons in the family, the husband would have to divorce a sterilized wife and get himself a new wife who might bear him sons.

What then would be the consequence to the woman following a divorce? She would be rejected from the family and lose whatever possessions she had, including custody of her own children, who would remain with their father and his family. Although this woman could remarry, she did not want to divorce the husband. She loves the family, and she especially did not want to lose custody of her daughters.

One participant intervened when this story was being told and asked, "What about her rights? Doesn't she have a right to decide for herself?" This rare use of "rights" language in China was seen as acceptable when it pertained to the right of a woman against her husband. There was no corresponding use of rights language to identify the rights of women or couples vis-à-vis the government.

This case was presented as having happened a long time ago. I asked whether it could still happen today and was told "yes, in some remote mountainous areas." Remote mountainous areas are ostensibly the places where traditional Chinese values respecting the authority of husbands and mothers-in-law still rule in the family. My guess is that the speaker did not want to admit to a visitor from the United States that similar things could occur in urban areas, as well, in modernized China.

Whether general principles are necessary or even useful is a topic of hot dispute among scholars in the field of bioethics. My own view is that without ethical principles as part of a framework, there can be no systematic way to justify ethical judgments. Opponents would reply that these principles are Western in origin and therefore cannot be used for justification across cultures. I maintain that without principles to serve as an ideal to strive for, there could be no concept of moral progress. Opponents would argue that the very notion of progress is a Western invention. To argue at length here for the relevance and importance of ethical principles would require endless digressions into the scholarly literature of bioethics. I plan to avoid such scholarly excursions and try to make my point with illustrative examples.

What I intend to show is that some things are relative, others are not. A convincing argument against ethical relativism need not conclude that *nothing* is relative, only that certain types of actions or practices—chiefly, those that violate human rights—are not. Because I reject the extremist version of ethical relativism, the task before me is to construct a plausible argument by way of rebuttal. One strategy toward that end will be to distinguish between explanation and justification. It is one thing to provide an explanation of why an individual or an entire culture holds certain beliefs and acts in certain ways. It is quite another thing to provide a justification for those beliefs and actions. Another strategy is to ask whether the consequences of traditional practices provide an objective basis for making ethical judgments. If a cultural practice produces manifest suffering or produces lifelong physical disability, there are good grounds for judging that practice to be ethically wrong. A well-known example is the historical practice in China of foot-binding women.

Ethical relativists question whether cross-cultural value judgments can ever be valid. If ethical norms are relative to time and place, it is a conceptual mistake, as well as a moral transgression, to pass judgments on other cultures. An even more radical step than making cross-cultural ethical judgments is for those outside a culture to seek to bring about changes in internal customs or traditions. Such actions were common among European colonial powers and Christian missionaries who saw themselves as undertaking the "white man's burden." These efforts eventually fell into disrepute as benighted attempts to "civilize the natives." The legitimacy of outside interference into the cultural or religious traditions of other societies today raises as much a political question as it does an ethical one. Not surprisingly, it is condemned as a new form of cultural imperialism or as an ethical version of "neocolonialism."[20]

So we need to separate the question of whether cross-cultural ethical judgments are legitimate and how they can be justified from the very different question of whether it is ethically permissible for outsiders to actively interfere with a culture's or nation's traditional practices. Even if there are some universal ethical principles capable of yielding transcultural moral judgments about a particular culture's traditional or religious practices, when, if ever, is it legitimate for outsiders to seek to change those practices? Defenders of ethical relativism use the term *ethical imperialism* to refer to situations in which one culture—usually Anglo-American or Western European—seeks to impose its ethical requirements on a less-developed country. If all such efforts are ethically suspect, then *ethical imperialism* is an apt term. But if ethical judgments of better or worse, more or less humane, can have cross-cultural validity, then *imperialism* is not a correct way to describe the transcultural imposition of values. A more accurate description would be *reform*. If the allegedly "superior" values express what are widely held to be human rights, there may exist an ethical obligation to try to bring about changes in countries or cultures where violations of those rights are occurring. The best way to do this—strategically as well as ethically—is to form alliances with people within those cultures who are seeking to bring about such changes.

The trouble is, the charge that something is a human rights violation has become so common and widespread that the term is in danger of losing its meaning and import. It is a mistake to assimilate all ethical values to the level of human rights. As the term implies, *human* rights are universal precisely because they are held to be fundamental moral requirements for treating all members of the species *Homo sapiens*. But to accept this view we must first agree that, in relevant respects, human beings everywhere are fundamentally alike. The view that all aspects of social life and culture are socially constructed must ultimately reject the idea that human beings everywhere are fundamentally alike and, with it, the notion that there are any human rights.

Notes

1. Richard A. Shweder, *Thinking Through Cultures* (Cambridge, MA: Harvard University Press, 1991), p. 14ff.

2. Christopher Clausen, "Welcome to Postculturalism," *The Key Reporter*, Vol. 62, No. 1 (1996), p. 2.

3. As quoted in Clausen, p. 2.

4. Shweder, p. 362, n. 8.

5. "Respect for persons" was introduced as a leading principle applied to research ethics in National Commission for the Protection of Human Subjects of Biomedical and Behavioral Research, *The Belmont Report: Ethical Principles and Guidelines for the Protection of Human Subjects of Research* (Washington, DC, 1979). The principle has been elaborated and applied to broader contexts in the four editions of Tom L. Beauchamp and James F. Childress, *Principles of Biomedical Ethics* (New York: Oxford University Press, 1979, 1983, 1989, 1994).

6. Diego Gracia, "The Intellectual Basis of Bioethics in Southern European Countries," *Bioethics*, Vol. 7, No. 2/3 (1993):97–107, p. 99.

7. For a detailed elaboration of this definition and the principle that follows from it, see Bruce Miller, "Autonomy," (ed.) Warren T. Reich, *Encyclopedia of Bioethics*, 2nd edition (New York: Macmillan, 1995), pp. 215–220.

8. Qiu Renzong, personal communication.

9. Ruth Macklin, "Universality of the Nuremberg Code," (eds.) George J. Annas and Michael A. Grodin, *The Nazi Doctors and the Nuremberg Code: Human Rights in Human Experimentation* (New York: Oxford University Press, 1992), pp. 240–257; Allen Buchanan, "Judging the Past: The Case of the Human Radiation Experiments," *Hastings Center Report*, Vol. 26, No. 3 (1996), pp. 25–30.

10. My visit to Nigeria was part of a project on ethics and reproductive health, which I conducted between 1992 and 1994 under a grant from the Ford Foundation.

11. I adopt the meaning of these principles as explicated in Beauchamp and Childress, 4th edition (1994).

12. The story was told to me during my visit to China as part of my Ford Foundation project by a program officer working for the Foundation.

13. Qiu Renzong, personal communication.

14. This took place during a visit to Mexico as part of my Ford Foundation project.

15. Anita Allen, "Abortion: Legal and Regulatory Issues," (ed.) Warren T. Reich, *Encyclopedia of Bioethics*, 2nd edition, Vol. 1 (New York: Macmillan, 1995), p. 22.

16. 60 U.S. 4795 (1992).

17. John A. Robertson, "*Casey* and the Resuscitation of *Roe v. Wade*," *Hastings Center Report*, Vol. 22, No. 5 (1992), pp. 24–28.

18. Material in this section about the Philippines is taken from interviews I conducted there as part of my Ford Foundation project.

19. María del Carmen Elu, "Abortion Yes, Abortion No, in Mexico," *Reproductive Health Matters*, No. 1 (1993):58–66, p. 59.

20. Soheir A. Morsy, "Safeguarding Women's Bodies: The White Man's Burden Medicalized," *Medical Anthropological Quarterly*, Vol. 5, No. 1 (1991), pp. 19–23.

2

Philosophers
and
Anthropologists
Debate

THE antirelativist assumes that ethical judgments do have objective validity or, at least, better or worse justifications. But philosophers, anthropologists, and other academics from a wide variety of fields in the postmodern era question that assumption. Especially when it comes to cross-cultural judgments, skepticism is widespread about whether any ethical justification is possible. This postmodern intellectual stance resurrects a long-standing philosophical contention: Cross-cultural ethical judgments are meaningless or impossible. Ethics has no objective basis. A counterpart exists in the field of anthropology, especially among those who base their ethical relativism on an underlying position, an "epistemological" or "cognitive" variety of relativism. That position maintains that the differences among cultures are much deeper than their customs, traditions, and values, extending to differences in the way in which the world is described and understood, as well as to fundamentally different modes of reasoning.

Anthropologists and Ethical Relativism

Debates among anthropologists about cultural and ethical relativism had an earlier wave and a more recent one. The earlier relativist position was a response by anthropologists to what they judged to be the prevailing cultural arrogance of Western European intellectuals. The current debate adopts features of the earlier one but goes further in also manifesting the widespread postmodern intellectual rejection of objective standards for making judgments in the arts, the social sciences, and even the natural sciences.

American anthropologists earlier in the twentieth century espoused cultural relativism as a moral force for tolerance.[1] This stance was a backlash against nineteenth century Social Darwinist theory and beliefs that prevailed at the time that Europe had a culture in all respects superior to that of other cultures. Cultural relativism emerged in reaction to the earlier theory of "cultural evolutionism, " a theory that held that human societies progressed in stages from "primitive" or "savage" to "modern." Cultural relativism was introduced in part to combat these racist, Eurocentric notions of progress.[2] The moral imperative of this movement was the requirement of tolerance.

A leading example can be found in the writings of the anthropologist Ruth Benedict. In *Patterns of Culture*, published in 1934, she wrote that "Morality differs in every society, and is a convenient term for socially approved habits." In this simple statement, Benedict made a subtle shift from a descriptive statement to a normative conclusion. The assumption underlying this shift is that whatever members of a society approve of is right, and whatever they disapprove of is wrong.

A few years later, other anthropologists argued from exactly the opposite moral imperative. Following the revelation of the horrors of the Holocaust after World War II, some anthropologists objected to the profession's adoption of cultural relativism, arguing that just as all human beings opposed the brutal treatment of Jews in Nazi Germany, a similar opposition might be called for in the many other kinds of discrimination and unfair practices found throughout the world.[3]

Unlike philosophers, who sit in their armchairs and write about ethical relativism, anthropologists who do fieldwork directly face cultural diversity in the groups they study and write about. These anthropologists generally adhere to the imperative adopted by their academic profession to respect the cultural differences they find and to avoid making value judgments that would inevitably reflect their own Western or developed-country biases. One discussion of the ethics of fieldwork begins with a little story designed to illustrate the anthropologists' dilemma.

"Over 1600 years ago, St. Augustine's mother was confronted with one of the dilemmas that faces nearly every anthropologist working in the field today. To St. Monica's question, 'At Rome they fast on Saturday, but not at Milan; which practice ought to be observed?', St Ambrose is reported to have replied, 'When I am at Milan I do as they do at Milan; but when I go to Rome, I do as Rome does."[4]

How does this story of St. Augustine's mother help to set the stage for the dilemma confronting anthropologists? Not at all, according to one philosopher: "Just as *de gustibus non disputandum* is not a maxim which applies to morality, neither is 'when in Rome do as the Romans do,' which is at best a principle of etiquette."[5] One reason, then, why anthropologists may not be in the best position to resolve the controversy over cultural and ethical relativism is that they typically fail to distinguish sharply between those customs and traditions that have ethical content and others that are matters of etiquette, ritual, or religion but have little or no relation to ethics.

An obvious reply is that what is considered a matter of ethics in one culture may not be in another. On this view, the very facts of cultural relativity make it impossible to use our twentieth century Western conception of what falls inside and outside the sphere of ethics and apply it to other cultures. Secular Western culture can normally distinguish between religion and ethics or between ethics and etiquette, but in some cultures there is no such line. The likely prospect that different conceptions of ethics exist in different cultures and that they may be incommensurable is one variety of the numerous types of ethical relativism.

Unfortunately for researchers in anthropology, their literature fails to give clear guidance about the obligations of fieldworkers. The opening paragraph of the American Association of Anthropology's Principles of Professional Responsibility (PPR) states that "anthropologists' first responsibility is to those whose lives and cultures they study." But what does this mean? As noted in a publication of that professional association:

> Anthropologists working in the field have witnessed female circumcision and infibulation [an extreme form of genital mutilation] in the Sudan, bride burnings in India, child abuse on the streets of Brazil and violence against women in cultures around the world. Some have invoked the principle of cultural relativity to justify a neutral stance as participant observers; others have adopted a more activist role. After weighing their personal and social values, advocates of 'when in Rome' base their involvement on the PPR: 'Should conflicts of interest arise, the interests of these people take precedence over other considerations.'[6]

This attempt to provide guidance simply restates the dilemma. Should the anthropologist interpret "the interests of these people" to mean preservation of the customs and traditions they practice whether or not those customs cause physical or other harms? Or does the proper interpretation allow for an assessment of the benefits and harms from outside the perspective of the culture itself? This requires making a distinction be-tween what people within a culture believe to be in their interests and what truly is in their interests, regardless of what they may believe.

Yet this very distinction is considered spurious by some cultural rela-tivists. The most extreme version of cultural relativism embodies a form of "cognitive" or "epistemological" relativism: It is impossible for anyone out-side a culture to fully understand practices and customs internal to a cul-ture. If it is impossible to understand "the other," it follows that it is illegiti-mate to judge "the other." A less extreme version of cultural relativism denies this extreme epistemological skepticism and allows that outsiders may come to understand the beliefs and practices of cultures other than their own. However, the imperative of ethical relativism remains firm: Judgments about what best serves the interest of the people should be left to members of that culture. Within the professional practice of anthro-pologists, it is left to researchers themselves to decide what constitutes an "interest of the people." Researchers in anthropology take positions on both sides of the issue.

The data from anthropology leave no doubt that the world contains enormous variations in cultural beliefs, customs, traditions, and practices. These data yield the rather simple descriptive thesis of cultural relativity or, as one anthropologist prefers to call this factual state of the world, "cul-tural diversity."[7] Beyond the key question for ethics—what follows from the facts of cultural diversity?—additional questions focus on our ability to gain a genuine understanding of cultures other than our own. Before we can get clear about what cultural relativism implies for ethics we might look to the anthropologists for an answer to the epistemological question: Do some cultures differ so much in their basic perception of the world, and employ such different conceptual categories, that cross-cultural un-derstanding is impossible to achieve?

Alas, we are not going to get the answer from anthropologists. This is because an anthropologist can be found in support of every variation, from the universalist persuasion to the most radical forms of relativism. On the extreme relativist end of the continuum is the position that all standards are culturally constituted, so there are no available *trans*cultural standards by which different cultures might be judged on a scale of merit or worth.[8]

This relativist position breaks down into two further variations. The first is "cognitive relativism," what philosophers would term "epistemological relativism." According to this view, the truth of any proposition is relative to the cognitive standards of the cultures in which it is embedded. "In short, all science is ethnoscience. Hence, since modern science is Western science, its truth claims (and canons of proof) are no less culturally relative than those of any other ethnoscience."[9] The second variation is full-blooded moral relativism: "The claims of ethical propositions are relative to the moral standards of the cultures in which they are embedded. . . . There are no universally acceptable standards by which [they] might be validly judged on a scale of relative merit or worth."[10]

The Chilean woman described in Chapter 1, who defended the beliefs of the indigenous people who engaged in ritual killing of their babies, was an adherent of this form of cognitive relativism. She referred to the judgment a Western scientist would make that failure to sacrifice babies does not cause droughts as "just a belief" on a par with the belief of the indigenous group that the drought they were experiencing was caused by the gods' anger at their omission of infant sacrifice. Another example is the belief in some societies where female genital mutilation is practiced that if the head of the emerging infant touches the mother's clitoris during childbirth, the child will become mentally retarded. In cultures that hold this belief, the justification for excision of the clitoris in women prior to marriage is the prevention of mental retardation in their children. A different belief relating to the same ritual is that if a woman's clitoris is not removed early in life, it will grow to the size of a man's penis, clearly an unacceptable anatomical feature in the female sex. Cognitive relativists would have to conclude that these "ethnoscientific" beliefs are as valid in the places where they are maintained as are our Western scientific beliefs about the causes of mental retardation and the anatomical development of genital organs.

Far along toward the other end of the continuum, some anthropologists have identified a number of different universals common to the human species. For example, Melford Spiro begins with the fact that humans are the product of biological (including behavioral) evolution. There is a causal relationship between a set of evolutionary biological characteristics and a set of universal social and cultural characteristics. From this it is reasonable to assume the existence of a set of universal psychological characteristics, such as pain avoidance, object constancy, attachment behavior, and others. Added to these universals is a third: the existence of strongly internalized cultural norms and values, which in turn cause emotionally painful reactions such as shame, guilt, and the lowering of self-esteem.[11] Spiro uses this brief inventory of cultural, social, and psychological universals to support his contention that it is only by rejecting human biological evolution that the premise of radical cultural pluralism—the incommensurability of cultures—can be sustained.

But it is not altogether clear what must follow from the identification of universal social and cultural characteristics. The anthropologist Melville Herskovits was one of the staunchest defenders of normative ethical relativism, yet he also claimed to identify certain cultural universals. He made a key distinction between absolutes and universals: "*Absolutes* are fixed, and, as far as convention is concerned, are not admitted to have variation, to differ from culture to culture, from epoch to epoch. *Universals*, on the other hand, are those least common denominators to be extracted from the range of variation that all phenomena of the natural or cultural world manifest."[12] The essence of this view is that universal forms that are found as human imperatives exist in all cultures, but there are no fixed contents to be found in any of these forms. This results in a seeming paradox, yet one that is readily understandable with sufficient explanation: "Morality is both universal and relative to the particular value system which gives it content."[13] If relativism and absolutism are not the only two alternatives, then an examination of universals may be promising. The concept of universals may point the way to a resolution of the impasse between those unacceptable extremes. After all, universality is what philosophers have claimed for ethical principles, despite the recent falling out of favor of such principles among bioethicists. If anthropologists have offered a plausible account of cultural universals, it may provide a bridge to a nonrelativistic ethics.

As is common in other contexts, people in this controversy disagree about what follows from premises on which they agree. The anthropologist Herskovits, who made such a nice distinction between universals and absolutes, remained a strong defender of normative ethical relativism. In contrast, other anthropologists use the data of anthropological universals to argue against the plausibility of extreme relativism.[14] These latter anthropologists reject the claims of their epistemological relativist colleagues, contending that the "human experience" of the alien peoples ethnographers study is comprehensible to them, so it can only be assumed that although culture, human nature, and the human mind are diverse enough, they are not all that diverse: "The characteristics which they share—the universal characteristics of culture, human nature, and the human mind—are at least as prominent as those in which they differ."[15]

One contemporary anthropologist counts himself among the distinct minority of his colleagues who seek to identify human universals and accord them great significance. Donald Brown contends that what we know about universals places clear limits on the cultural relativism that anthropologists have described and promoted.[16] Brown provides a heterogeneous catalogue of human universals, some of which appear to be inherent in human nature while others are cultural conventions that are distributed universally. Universals rooted in human neurobiology include the "formal" deep structure of language put forth by Noam Chomsky and the processes involved in human bonding described by the anthropologist Robin Fox.[17] Other types of universals are considered as "frameworks" or "models" existing in every culture, for example, "the men usually exercise control" and "primary kin do not mate with each other."[18] Still other types of universals demonstrated by empirical studies are facial expressions that convey emotions and facial recognition, thereby giving individuals the ability to recognize kin. The implications for ethics of the universals identified by anthropologists are not immediately evident, but they suggest at the very least that, despite the superficial diversity of cultures, similar underlying structures and frameworks can be found.

A necessary step in attempting to apply ethical principles to customs and traditions is to distinguish between practices that have moral content and those that are morally neutral. This project is, of course, complicated by cross-cultural differences that could lead people from Western culture to consider as morally neutral actions or practices that people within another culture believe to have moral significance. Remarking on the diversity of beliefs, desires, and practices that research has uncovered, one anthropologist offers a short list of the things we can observe out there in the world of human beings:

> People hunting for witches, exorcising demons, propitiating dead ancestors, sacrificing animals to hungry gods, sanctifying temples, waiting for messiahs, scapegoating their sins, consulting the stars, decoding their dreams, flagellating themselves in public, prohibiting the eating of pork (or dog, or beef or all swarming things except locusts, crickets, and grasshoppers), wandering on pilgrimage from one dilapidated shrine to the next, abstaining from sex on the day of the full moon, refusing to be in the same room with their wife's elder sister, matting their hair with cow dung, isolating women during menstruation, seeking salvation by meditating naked in a cave for several years, and so on and on.[19]

These examples of diverse cultural beliefs and practices illustrate the descriptive thesis of cultural relativity—the fact that cultures differ from one another, sometimes radically. The nagging question remains: What, if anything, follows for ethics from the facts of cultural relativity? Some of the items on this short list involve no harm to self or others, whereas others pose some risk of damaging physical or psychological consequences to the agent or those who are affected. I hold the view that moral judgments apply only to those actions or practices that have consequences for others. This leaves actions like decoding dreams, flagellating oneself (in public or private), dietary restrictions, and meditating in caves beyond the pale of moral judgment. Self-regarding actions may be wise or foolish, beneficial or harmful, prudent or imprudent, but they are not, strictly speaking, candidates for moral judgment.

There are three standard objections to this view of ethics. The first objection is the "no man is an island" criticism (in its politically correct version, "no person is an island"). Everything we do affects others, this critique maintains, so actions that appear to have consequences only for the person who performs them will inevitably affect others. Causing physical harm to oneself by self-flagellation has at least psychological consequences for those near and dear to the flagellator and may affect others by requiring

nursing care during the healing process; the person whose dreams are de-
coded may alter behavior in ways likely to affect others; unless one is a her-
mit, dietary restrictions will be imposed on the one who buys and prepares
the food and will likely restrict the options for others in the household; and
so on. I accept this criticism with the reply that it is an empirical matter, to
be decided on a case-by-case basis when an action affects only the person
who performs it and when it also affects others. It is likely that the vast majority of human actions in every culture affect persons besides the agent.
In that case, all those actions are subject to moral review.

The second objection contends that it is a mistaken or narrow view of
morality to maintain that ethical judgments are only proper when a person's actions have consequences for others. "Duties to oneself" is a Kantian category adapted to everyday conversation in remarks like "I owe it to
myself to." But this is not a genuine judgment of obligations to oneself.
People make such statements in attempts to justify their own self-interested actions. Because self-interested actions need not always be selfish,
the utterance is not invariably self-serving in a way that is ethically suspect.
People do, of course, have certain responsibilities to themselves, such as
the responsibility to care for one's health. Still, the main purpose of a
moral system is to set rules and ethical standards for people's conduct toward others. The natural inclination to look out for one's own interests is
in no need of the judgments and sanctions of a moral system.

The third objection is more radical than the first two. It maintains
that the concept of a person is itself socially or culturally constructed, and
therefore it is a mistake to employ our Western, individualistic concept of a
person and assume that it applies to non-Western cultures or is understandable to them. As soon as the terms *socially constructed* and *culturally
constructed* appear, we know we are in the postmodern landscape, territory
in which there is little objective reality except (perhaps) the physical world
around us. If the Western or "Eurocentric" conception of ethics is narrowly individualistic, so too is the concept of a person on which our familiar ethical formulations rest. This view not only has implications for the
universality of ethics; it also implies an epistemological relativism in how
people come to learn about life that would make intercultural communications and understanding next to impossible.

It is no simple task to try to apply the varieties of relativism and universalism to actual examples from different cultures. One anthropologist provides an example that is intended to acknowledge the existence of cultural universals and at the same time to illustrate that it is compatible with one species of relativism. The cultural group in this example is the Oriya Brahmans in India.[20] While people in this culture disapprove of kicking a dog that is sleeping on a street, they do not disapprove of beating a wife who goes to the movies without the husband's permission. Kicking the dog would count as an "arbitrary assault," whereas beating an errant wife would not. Furthermore, Oriya Brahmans disapprove of some treatments they consider unfair, such as nepotism, cutting in line, and a hotel rule that excludes invalids from the dining hall. Yet other practices they consider fair, for example, for the son to inherit far more than the daughter. Therefore, the anthropologist concludes, "the appeal to some small set of common abstract principles (justice, harm, protecting the vulnerable, etc.) does not help us understand or predict which cases will be seen as alike or different." The analogy goes like this: Beating a wife who goes to the movies without her husband's permission is roughly equivalent to corporal punishment for a soldier who leaves the military base without permission.

The "universals" in this example are the "abstract" formal principle of justice, "treat like cases alike," and the prohibition against arbitrary assault. Oriya Brahmans, like Westerners, consider it wrong to kick a dog that is sleeping on the street. In both cultures this act is an instance of arbitrary assault. On the other hand, while Oriya Brahmans do not disapprove of beating "black and blue" a wife who goes to the movies without the husband's permission, Western culture disapproves of such acts. The cultural difference lies in the traditions of the culture that determine whether beating a wife is, like kicking a dog, an example of an arbitrary assault (the Western view); or whether beating a wife is, like corporal punishment for a private in the army who leaves the military base without permission, a justified physical assault (the Oriya Brahman view).

The difference between the Oriya Brahman view and the Western view is not simply one of judging different actions to be ethically permissible or prohibited. It is also a question of which similarities or differences are morally relevant in applying the principle "arbitrary physical assault is wrong." A simple comparison of the acts themselves could lead to the conclusion that the Oriya Brahmans value dogs more than wives because it is impermissible to kick the former animals when it is doing nothing but sleeping yet permissible to beat up the latter for doing nothing but going to the movies without the permission of husbands. But once we understand that the relationship between husbands and wives in the institution of marriage is in relevant respects like the hierarchical structure in the military, then we can understand how the Oriya Brahmans can approve of husbands beating up on wives who neglect to ask permission to leave the house: The wives have broken a rule. It does not matter that Westerners might also disapprove of corporal punishment of military subordinates; what matters is understanding the cultural institutions that confer similarity on wives and privates in the army.

This is a perfect example of the difference between explanation of a cultural phenomenon and justification of it. Before becoming enlightened about the way Oriya Brahmans view similarities and differences between physical assaults that are arbitrary and those that are not, we would misunderstand the grounds on which they disapprove of kicking dogs but not of beating wives. How should this new understanding of the way Oriya Brahmans apply the formal principle "treat like cases alike" affect our Western propensity to condemn that culture's condoning wife beating? My answer is: Not in the least.

We now have an explanation, but it still does not serve as a justification. What needs to be justified in the next step is an institution of marriage that embodies a military-like hierarchy, one in which one party has absolute authority over the other and that authority includes administering physical beatings for failure to adhere to the rules of permission that govern subordinates. The relativist holds that marriage in the West and marriage among the Oriya Brahmans are two different social institutions. Western societies are more egalitarian, Indian society much less so. Even in an egalitarian Western society some institutions, such as the military, are hierarchical and distinctly inegalitarian. It would be just as absurd, the relativist would contend, to say that the United States Army should be a democratically run, egalitarian institution as to insist that the institution of marriage among the Oriya Brahmans should grant wives a status equal to husbands.

This conclusion requires that we accept social institutions as they are, without the possibility or desirability of change. But we reject slavery today because our more enlightened moral views prohibit treating human beings of whatever race, ethnicity, or social class like animals or, even worse, as inanimate property. At least on paper, we have reformed hierarchical institutions like the military and penal institutions to prohibit physical brutality and torture because we believe those practices to be unacceptably inhumane, if not violations of human rights. To argue that once we understand the Oriya Brahman institution of marriage we are somehow compelled to accept its features buys into the view that "whatever is, is right." This form of moral nihilism is not worth discussing in a book devoted to ethics.

Philosophers and Ethical Relativism

Philosophers as well as anthropologists have carried on debates about ethical relativism for a good part of the twentieth century. It is clear from reading the literature in these two academic disciplines that few people in either field are acquainted with the arguments and distinctions made by those in the other. Each has its own distinctions, its own radical and moderate spokespersons, and its own internecine wars. The anthropologists have empirical data on their side, while philosophers tend to rely on arguments that are mounted with precision and rigor.

The philosophical debate begins with an extreme and rather simplistic version. One prominent philosopher refers to the "vulgar" form of relativism, which he characterizes as consisting of three propositions: (1) "right" means "right for a given society"; (2) "right for a given society" is to be understood in a functionalist sense; and therefore (3) it is wrong for people in one society to condemn, criticize, or interfere with the values of another society. The thesis of ethical relativism, characterized by these three propositions, is logically inconsistent. The third proposition states that it is *wrong* for people in one society to condemn or interfere with the values of another society. But the first proposition does not allow use of the term *wrong* in this nonrelative sense, that is, outside its meaning within a particular culture.[21] While this "vulgar" position contends that morality is relative, at the same time it takes a nonrelative stance with regard to the moral requirement of toleration.

It is possible that some unsophisticated people have actually held this so-called "vulgar" form of relativism. But even in a less vulgar form, if ethical relativism were a logically coherent position, it would not only follow that members of one culture or historical era could never criticize on moral grounds the socially approved practices of another time or place; there could also be no such thing as moral progress. Abolition of slavery could not be seen as a moral victory, but only as political change. The eighth amendment to the U.S. Constitution, prohibiting cruel and unusual punishment, could be viewed only as a product of the beliefs of the framers of the Bill of Rights. Granting social and economic equality to women and to blacks, thereby overturning centuries of injustice, could only be viewed as peculiarities of mid-twentieth century political movements.

But if this extreme version of ethical relativism is flawed and therefore unacceptable, what are the alternatives? At the opposite extreme are the claims of ethical absolutism. This alternative has the unfortunate consequence of abandoning the frying pan of ethical relativism for the fire of ethical absolutism. One defense of absolutism begins with the claim that any form of ethical relativism is equivalent to radical subjectivism, which reduces to the position that there does not exist a moral standard anywhere that is binding upon people against their will. The very possibility of moral valuation disappears.[22]

The absolutist, on the contrary, believes in the existence of a single universal moral standard, which yields commands that all people have an obligation to obey.[23] The obvious problem with this version of ethical absolutism is that no one has articulated such a universal morality or shown the plausibility of an ethical theory that can provide a basis for a universal morality. The absolutist must fall back on the idle hope that perhaps such a theory will be found tomorrow. A counterpart to the "vulgar" form of ethical relativism, this extreme defense of ethical absolutes might be termed "crude" absolutism.

A more sophisticated philosophical attempt begins with a distinction between ultimate moral principles and specific moral standards or rules.[24] Both can be called *norms*, but relativists tend to overlook this distinction. On this multilevel view, the key to rebutting ethical relativism lies in understanding that an ultimate moral principle can be consistent with a variety of specific standards and rules that can be found in the moral codes of different societies.

Examples of such specific moral standards are specific rules of conduct, such as "Do not tell lies for one's own advantage," which prescribe how people ought or ought not to act. These specific standards or rules are on a different level from ultimate moral principles. The latter are not "moral absolutes" but, rather, universal propositions about the conditions under which a standard is to be used to judge any person or action. One prominent example of an ultimate moral principle is the utilitarian principle that right actions or practices are those that tend to produce an increase in overall happiness or welfare and a decrease in overall unhappiness or suffering.

When a general principle like this is applied to different societies, it is evident that a specific standard or rule that increases people's happiness in one culture will not increase, but rather decrease, people's happiness in another. A long-standing (if overused) example is letting elderly people die when they can no longer contribute to economic production in societies characterized by extreme scarcity. When that practice is necessary for the survival of everyone else, it conforms to the principle of utility. In a society of abundance, however, old people can easily be supported when they are no longer productive and their continued existence does not threaten the lives or well-being of others. According to this analysis, letting old, nonproductive members of society die would be ethically right in the former society and ethically wrong in the latter. Remarkably, however, the notion that there is "a duty to die" appears to be gaining prominence today in the most affluent society in the world.[25]

A multilevel view of ethics makes it possible to distinguish between ultimate moral principles and specific rules or codes of conduct, a distinction that is necessary for reaching some sort of accommodation between the unacceptable extremes of vulgar relativism and crude absolutism. But the analysis stops short of another foundational problem in ethics: how to determine which of several ultimate moral principles to accept in cases where they conflict. The principle of utility, mentioned in the above example to illustrate the consistency of having a single ultimate principle while allowing for different specific rules of conduct, is not the only ultimate ethical principle. Another leading candidate is "respect for persons," a form of the Kantian categorical imperative mandating that people are to be treated as ends, never merely as means to the ends of others. Resolving this foundational problem in philosophical ethics need not concern us here, since it is not required for drawing some conclusions about cultural and ethical relativism.

A problem with the multilevel view that must be addressed, however, is the difficulty of justifying particular ethical judgments by appealing to an ultimate ethical principle like the principle of utility. Defenders of female genital mutilation contend that the practice is ethically acceptable in their culture because it is a deeply rooted tradition that binds women together, renders women marriageable (whereas uncircumcised women are not marriageable), and therefore contributes to the harmony and overall well-being of the society. Critics of this ritual, from within and outside the societies in which it is practiced, use the principle of utility to justify the opposite ethical judgment: Female genital mutilation is ethically unacceptable because it causes extreme pain in girls and women at the time it is performed, it often leads to serious and lifelong physical ailments, including infertility, and sometimes results in severe infection, hemorrhage, and death. The contradictory ethical judgments resulting from this analysis are not a function of ethical relativism but, rather, stem from the difficulty of measuring happiness, well-being, disability, and death as required in attempts to apply the utilitarian principle.

Cultural Universals and Ethical Principles

It is time to review the distinctions among different types of relativism and try to clarify what each version maintains. So far we have descriptive relativism, a view that emerges from the facts of cultural variability or diversity. This is an empirical generalization drawn from observations of different cultures. No one denies the truth of this descriptive thesis, but disagreements begin with the question: What follows from the facts of cultural diversity?

Next is normative ethical relativism in its simple and extreme form: "Right" and "wrong" are totally culture-dependent concepts, and there is no meaningful or objective way of making moral judgments outside one's own cultural setting. The "vulgar," self-contradictory version of this extreme view adds the proposition that "it is wrong to make cross-cultural ethical judgments." Without the addition of the self-contradictory statement, extreme ethical relativism is the prevailing postmodern view.

Then there is the position termed *cognitive* or *epistemological* relativism, held by some anthropologists, according to which the ways of knowing and the canons of justification and proof vary from one culture to another, so cross-cultural understanding of alien customs and morality is impossible. Some defenders of normative ethical relativism base their position on this underlying cognitive relativism, but ethical relativism can stand alone without this epistemological underpinning.

Next we have the opposite extreme, the *crude* version of absolutism: There exists a set of moral commands, obedience to which is obligatory on all people, whether they know it or not, whatever they feel, and whatever their customs may be. A more refined version of absolutism is a form of "natural law" theory of morality. According to the predominant Roman Catholic teachings, "natural law" is God given and contains moral absolutes.

Next we have the array of views somewhere in the middle, beginning with the philosophical distinction between specific moral standards and ultimate moral principles. Normative ethical relativism may be the correct way to characterize the variety of specific moral standards throughout the world, but it does not apply to ultimate moral norms that underlie this large variety of specific rules. According to this view, some things are relative (specific moral standards) while others are not (ultimate moral principles).

Another middle-ground philosophical account begins with the question, "Assuming that cultural relativity is a fact, what follows for ethics?" and goes on to reply:

What follows depends in part upon just what turns out to be relative. . . . There are at least ten quite different things of interest to the ethicist that the anthropologist might discover to be relative to culture: mores, social institutions, human nature, acts, goals, value experiences, moral emotions, moral concepts, moral judgments and moral reasoning.[26]

This intriguing suggestion calls for providing a detailed analysis of the above 10 items in the context of an anthropological study. If human universals can be identified, as some anthropologists contend, then at least some of the items on this list will not be relative to culture.

The anthropologists' middle-ground position applied to ethics relies on positing the existence of at least some cultural universals. One anthropologist's version begins with the claim that relativism does not preclude the possibility of cross-cultural universals discovered through empirical research.[27] A further elucidation of this view states:

A cross-cultural universal provides the standard for judging right and wrong. . . . The difference between universals and absolutes permits us to distinguish the relativist approach from that of the natural law theorist on the important issue of social change. Natural law posits immutable moral principles whose origin resides in nature. By contrast, cross-cultural universals are moral principles whose source is found in cultural ideas that may evolve.[28]

The way out of the impasse between the two extremes appears to lie in the quest for universals: both the anthropologists' and the philosophers' versions. Cultural universals, as discovered by anthropologists, and ethical universals, as described by philosophers, have to be somehow brought together to combat the various versions of relativism. The only obvious way to do this is to rescue ethical principles from the attack they have been subjected to by philosophers, bioethicists, and some anthropologists who have joined the battle against "principlism." The attack on principles and the way it has been mounted in the bioethics literature misinforms scholars and writers from other fields who take their cues from people inside the field.

Here is one statement in an article by two anthropologists misled in this way: "Recent developments in bioethical theory have challenged the deductive model of ethical reasoning, which proceeds from abstract principles (as do both cultural relativism and universalism) to moral judgments."[29] What is especially remarkable about this critique of principles is that it appears in the context of a discussion about cultural relativism and universalism. How could anthropologists get the idea that a bioethical methodology that employs ethical principles "proceeds from them alone in a deductive process"? Nowhere can one find in the bioethics literature that embraces fundamental principles anything resembling an argument in deductive logic except, perhaps, as a parody of ethical reasoning.

These anthropologists who join bioethicists in rejecting principles imply a preference for other methodologies in bioethics that avoid the alleged deductive method: "Casuistry, or contextual, case-based reasoning may consider moral principles, but does not proceed from them alone in a deductive process. Rather, contextual elements like historical and cultural issues, power relations, and responsibility are important factors to consider."[30] This is a fuzzy formulation. What does it mean for other forms of ethical reasoning to "consider moral principles"? When we are urged to "consider" these other important factors, how is their consideration supposed to help us reach a conclusion? The vagueness of this sort of critique almost makes one long for a deductive argument.

Ethical analysis of individual cases or specific situations *always* proceeds by relating the facts and circumstances to whatever ethical judgment or conclusion is eventually reached. How, for example, could one begin to apply the principle of nonmaleficence or beneficence without examining the facts: actual or probable harms (physical, psychological, or social) produced by research on human subjects and the potential benefits to the research subjects themselves or to future patients? What has the patients' rights movement, the emphasis on respect for the patient's autonomy, and the implementation of informed consent been about if not a recognition of the unequal power relations between doctors and patients? When it comes to cultural issues, bioethics in the multicultural United States has always grappled with the particular circumstances of religious or ethnic minorities in questioning whether respect for autonomy should permit Jehovah's Witnesses to refuse relatively low-risk, life-saving blood transfusions that doctors say would violate their beneficence-based obligations; whether a pregnant woman who comes from a culture opposed to cutting may refuse a cesarean section deemed necessary to preserve the life or health of her fetus; whether the obligation to respect the autonomy of the patient should override the customs of an immigrant family in which the patriarch makes all decisions and insists that physicians not converse with his wife about her treatment options. In short, it is impossible to consider clinical ethics or health policy ethics without paying attention to context, cultural issues, power relations, and all the contextual elements these and other anthropologists identify as relevant.

The oft-heard criticism that the principles of respect for persons, beneficence, and justice are "abstract" and therefore fail to adequately take into account the social context and specific features of problematic situations is absurd. Of course principles are "abstract" in form. That is their virtue. They would not otherwise count as *principles* but would instead be specific rules or instructions in a code of conduct. The unavoidable and inherent abstractness of the principles themselves implies nothing whatsoever about how they are to be applied to personal, social, or professional situations. To apply any "abstract" ethical principle it is first necessary to look at the social context, to take account of who stands to be affected and in what ways, and to factor in a large array of particular circumstances. There is no algorithm, no "deductive" procedure for doing that.

Another peculiar assumption of these critics is that ethical principles do not require elucidation and interpretation. That, too, is absurd. The ways of understanding and implementing general principles are numerous and can take different forms in different contexts, countries, or cultures. The bioethical principle of *beneficence*, or, more generally, the utilitarian principle on which it relies, is a case in point. Beneficence embodies the commonsense notion that right actions and practices are those that result in a balance of beneficial consequences over ones that are harmful. Although the statement of the principle itself is "abstract," its concrete application requires considerable empirical data and a knowledge of the particular context in which it is applied.

One anthropologist who engages in clinical ethics hails the recent moves by some of her colleagues away from the approach that uses ethical principles to analyze dilemmas or problems. Likening the "new thinking in bioethics" to the traditional stance of anthropology, she describes the difference between philosophy and anthropology. She observes that whereas anthropology has a long tradition of examining values, anthropologists most certainly have not made moral judgments of the cultural institutions and practices they have studied. Anthropologists recognize that the definition of a medical dilemma and its ethical resolution are intertwined with cultural factors that influence behavior related to health and illness.

These observations are surely true, but where do they leave us? What follows from the deliberate omission of moral judgments by anthropologists conducting their work? Does it mean that philosophers who engage in transcultural studies should also refrain from making moral judgments? Or that the movement in recent bioethics toward ethnography shows that ethicists have now come to see the light? We have to bear in mind two salient points: first, that the aims and purposes of anthropology are quite different from those of normative ethics; second, if we deny the legitimacy of making cross-cultural ethical judgments we are doomed to accept the status quo: "whatever is, is right."

Yet it is abundantly clear that the anthropologist who acts in the capacity of an ethics consultant in her own culture *does* make ethical judgments at least implicitly, if not explicitly. She worries (quite rightly) about ethicists who do consultations in the medical setting being "co-opted" by the biomedical system. She reminds us that the status differentials between physicians and all other parties is considerable, leading to the danger that the ethics consultant will serve as a "powerbroker" or mediator between two opposing parties. In a setting in which the parties to a dispute are not equal, and where the ethics consultant does not call the shots, the danger of co-optation is greatest. As a result, she notes, the patients' values and goals for medical treatment may end up being compromised.[32]

The term *cooptation* is hardly the ethically neutral language of the descriptive anthropologist. It is a language infused with value judgments. The anthropologist–ethicist's worry that the patient's values may become subordinated to those of the biomedical system—an entirely appropriate concern—exhibits her clear value bias in favor of patient autonomy and self-determination. We are left wondering whether her overall account is consistent. On the one hand, she contrasts the methods of anthropology with those of philosophical ethics, admonishing the latter discipline for relying in its value judgments on standards of moral rectitude and framing problems in the language of rights and autonomy. On the other hand, when she dons the hat of clinical ethicist, she defends the importance of respect for patients' values and beliefs and their goals for medical treatment, worrying that the ethics consultant may be co-opted by the power of the medical profession.

An explanation for this apparent inconsistency might be the following. When in their own culture, anthropologists may make value judgments; but when studying another, different culture, they must refrain from making value judgments. This explanation is consistent with a version of ethical relativism that says it is permissible for people to make value judgments within their own cultural milieu, but not cross-culturally. This is because all values are culturally dependent or, in the currency of the day, "socially constructed." Although this explanation dispels the inconsistency, it bears an unhappy consequence for the prospects of reform in the way medicine is practiced in many developing countries. In those places, physicians have a disregard for patients' values and beliefs and their goals for medical treatment. No ethics consultants are available, even to run the risk of being co-opted. Physicians rule the medical domain with virtually absolute authority.

Now, the anthropologist can either claim that those are the cultural values, and we in the West must accept them and refrain from criticizing them, or else maintain that patients in developing countries deserve as much respect as patients are (or ought to be) given in the United States. To refrain from criticizing the way doctors treat patients in other countries is to acknowledge that a form of second-class citizenship for patients is ethically acceptable if they happen to live in a Third World country. On the other hand, to maintain that patients deserve respect for their values, wherever they happen to live, is to admit the existence of at least some cross-cultural universals. Respect for patients' values and goals for medical treatment is an instance of the broader ethical principle of respect for persons. Like it or not, critics of ethical principles end up employing them, at least implicitly, if they make any ethical judgments at all.

A defense of ethical principles in the international arena must begin with several caveats. The first caveat is not to commit the genetic fallacy. Just because certain ethical principles were first articulated in Western philosophy does not mean that such principles apply only in Western or Northern countries. Just because certain ethical principles first found expression in governmental regulations applied to research in the United States does not mean that they are not equally relevant to the regulatory framework elsewhere. The origins of ethical principles are one thing; their domain of applicability is another.

The second caveat is a reminder not to confuse the universality of principles with the quite different notion of an "absolutist ethics." *Universality* refers to the scope of applicability of ethical principles, whereas *absolutism* implies an exceptionless set of immutable moral rules or prescriptions. The four principles of bioethics (respect for persons, beneficence, nonmaleficence, and justice)[33] are very general and require interpretation in light of relevant empirical facts and contexts before they can be applied. Indeed, the principles are so general that they have been criticized as being "empty." They lack specific content. In contrast, "moral absolutes" are ethical judgments stating that certain types of action are "always" obligatory or "never" permissible, such as a rule-bound, absolute prohibition of lying.

A third caveat is that principles are necessary but not sufficient for a rich ethical analysis of human behavior. Those who argue for the importance of context in making moral judgments are correct in their insistence, but they are mistaken if they hold that context is all that is needed. They are also mistaken, as I have already noted, in thinking that principles can be used in an ethical analysis without bringing in facts and background circumstances.

Some ethicists stress the superiority of "narrative," which is supposed to provide a deep understanding of particular situations by supplying a history and set of experiences from which the people involved derive their beliefs and values. While I agree that such narratives can enrich ethical inquiry and deepen our understanding, narrative alone cannot do the work of justification. Narratives may be valuable for the purpose of *explanation* of why people have the beliefs, attitudes, values, or sentiments they hold;

but explanation is not *justification*, and the two should not be confused.

A case in point is the treatment of widows according to Hindu custom in parts of India. According to one Indian sociologist, to be a Hindu widow even today is to suffer "social death."[34] Hindu brides marry into their husbands' families and largely abandon ties to their own families. When the husband dies, the widow is left entirely dependent on her in-laws. If a woman is unfortunate enough to become a widow at a young age, she may be forced to work as an unpaid servant for her mother-in-law for decades to come. For their part, the in-laws do not want the financial responsibility of caring for another individual who does not support herself, so many widows are shoved out of the house or leave on their own accord. Widows thus face the miserable options of either remaining in indentured servitude to their dead husbands' families or leaving the home for a life of begging or prostitution. The historical tradition was for widows to be forced to have sex with men in their deceased husbands' families, and this prospect remains even today for some of the younger widows. These practices have their roots in ancient Hindu texts, in which mandate "the avoidance of widows." Remarriage is ruled out, as it would dishonor the family. Learning that the source of the contemporary treatment of widows lies in ancient Hindu texts and in the continuity of historical tradition does much to explain today's practice but offers nothing by way of justification. The principle of nonmaleficence provides a basis for judging the treatment of widows in these parts of India to be harmful, degrading, and, therefore, morally wrong.

My experience in carrying out international projects in bioethics has shown that general ethical principles can be very useful, not only for cross-cultural communications but also for helping colleagues in non-Western or developing countries to formulate persuasive arguments against traditional customs or restrictive laws that they themselves are seeking to change in their own societies. In countries where the only language of ethics is the specific code of morality enunciated by the dominant church or religious authority, people who reject the prescriptions or prohibitions of that code find it useful to have available a secular language of ethics.

At several meetings in Mexico devoted to ethics and reproductive health, I used the principles of respect for persons, beneficence, and justice in analyses of various problems participants brought to the table. Participants in those meetings expressed gratitude at being given a new set of tools with which to mount ethical arguments against their opponents — religious leaders and politicians unwilling to decriminalize abortion in Mexico. Women's health advocates acknowledged that the hierarchy of the Catholic Church would not be convinced by secular arguments that use the "respect for persons" principle to justify removing prohibitions on contraceptives, voluntary sterilization, or elective abortion. But those seeking reform said that respect for persons, beneficence, and distributive justice provide an alternative ethical vocabulary that can be valuable. People who are confused or "on the fence" about issues like contraception and abortion and who know only the official language of morality enunciated by the Catholic Church confront those dilemmas in a new way when they are provided with general principles they see as applicable to broad areas of social and political life.

In many parts of the world, the doctrine of informed consent to treatment is still unknown or, even when known, is not adhered to in practice. Informed consent is thought to be a "Western custom" in some countries, and its purpose is misunderstood as that of protecting doctors against lawsuits brought by their patients. At meetings in the Philippines, China, India, Bangladesh, Ivory Coast, and Nigeria, I made presentations on informed consent, arguing that it is not a North American or European *custom*, but rather an ethically necessary feature of the physician–patient relationship and the researcher–subject encounter justified by the principle of "respect for persons." Many participants in those meetings had never before considered informed consent as anything other than a Western custom in which patients or research subjects put their signature on a piece of paper. But they had no trouble recognizing that in their countries physicians often treat patients with disrespect and maintain a supremely paternalistic medical practice. Informed consent gained new meaning when put in the context of showing respect for persons by communicating with patients about proposed treatments and asking their permission to invade their bodies. It is impossible to justify the ethical requirement of informed consent to treatment or research by telling stories, however rich and nuanced they may be, or by appealing to communitarian interests. To distinguish between mere customs or cultural traditions, on the one hand, and practices that can be justified ethically, on the other, we need to use principles.

Another widely held assumption is that traditions embody cultural or other values that must always be respected. In Nigeria and in Egypt, I met with women and men seeking to combat the practice of female genital mutilation. The response to their efforts by defenders of this custom is that they have become dupes of Western cultural imperialism; they are failing to show respect for tradition in their own culture. But any custom or tradition can be examined and challenged on ethical grounds. To do so, one needs to have general principles that can supply a justification for rejecting or abandoning a long-established tradition. The opponents of female genital mutilation whom I met in Egypt and Nigeria seized upon relevant principles of bioethics as a helpful strategy in replying to those who defend custom and tradition simply because it is part of the cultural heritage.

It remains true that some societies do not recognize democratic institutions and deny that individuals have rights altogether, whether against the state or other powerful agencies. An appeal to principles such as "respect for persons" or "justice" will not work in those settings. This is a reminder that we must start with at least some shared, fundamental values. As we approach the year 2000, it is evident that there exist in the world some shared, fundamental values. The concept of human rights is intended to embrace such values. The fact that some governments contend that human rights is a Western invention, or that it is a form of ethical imperialism to impose that Western concept on cultures with a different tradition, does not demonstrate that there is no such thing as human rights. Rather it serves to remind us that those who hold power seek to maintain that power, sometimes by any means possible.

Notes

1. Sandra D. Lane and Robert A. Rubinstein, "Judging the Other: Responding to Traditional Female Genital Surgeries," *Hastings Center Report*, Vol. 26, No. 3 (1996), pp. 31–40.

2. Alison D. Renteln, "Relativism and the Search for Human Rights," *American Anthropologist* Vol. 90 (1988), p. 57.

3. Lane and Rubinstein, p. 32.

4. Susan N. Skomal, "The Ethics of Fieldwork," *Anthropology Newsletter*, Vol. 34, No. 7, (October 1993).

5. Bernard Williams, *Morality: An Introduction to Ethics* (New York: Harper Torchbooks, 1972), p. 24.

6. *Anthropology Newsletter*, Vol. 34, No. 7 (October 1993).

7. Melford Spiro, "Cultural Relativism and the Future of Anthropology," *Cultural Anthropology* Vol. I (1986), pp. 259–286.

8. Spiro, p. 260.

9. Spiro, p. 260.

10. Spiro, p. 260.

11. Spiro, p. 266.

12. Renteln, p. 66, citing Melville Herskovits, *Cultural Relativism: Perspectives in Cultural Pluralism* (New York: Random House, 1972), pp. 31–32.

13. Paul Rabinow, "Humanism as Nihilism: The Bracketing of Truth and Seriousness in American Cultural Anthropology," (eds.) Norma Haan, Robert N. Bellah, Paul Rabinow, and William M. Sullivan, *Social Science as Moral Inquiry* (New York: Columbia University Press, 1983), p. 58.

14. See, for example, Melford Spiro and Alison Renteln, cited above.

15. Spiro, pp. 268–269.

16. Donald E. Brown, *Human Universals* (Philadelphia: Temple University Press, 1991), p. vii.

17. Brown, pp. 42–47.

18. Brown, p. 47.

19. Richard A. Shweder, *Thinking Through Cultures* (Cambridge, MA: Harvard University Press, 1991), p. 30.

20. Richard A. Shweder, "Ethical Relativism: Is There a Defensible Version?" *Ethos*, Vol. 18, No. 2 (1990), pp. 205–217.

21. Bernard Williams, *Morality: An Introduction to Ethics* (New York: Harper & Row, 1972), pp. 20–21. In later writings, Williams takes the view that there is truth in relativism. See "The Truth in Relativism" in his *Moral Luck* (Cambridge University Press: London, 1981), pp. 132–143.

22. Walter T. Stace, "Ethical Relativity," (ed.) Paul W. Taylor, *Problems of Moral Philosophy* (Encino, CA: Dickenson Publishing Co., 1972), pp. 51–65.

23. Stace, p. 57.

24. An example is the following account provided by Paul W. Taylor, *Principles of Ethics: An Introduction* (Encino, CA: Dickenson Publishing Co., 1975).

25. See, for example, John Hardwig, "Is There a Duty To Die?" *Hastings Center Report* Vol. 27, No. 2 (1997), pp. 34–42.

26. Carl Wellman, "The Ethical Implications of Cultural Relativity," (ed.)

Paul W. Taylor, Problems of Moral Philosophy (Encino, CA: Dickenson Publishing Co., 1972), p. 74.

27. Renteln, p. 56.

28. Renteln, p. 66.

29. Lane and Rubinstein, p. 31.

30. Lane and Rubinstein, p. 31.

31. Patricia A. Marshall, "Anthropology and Bioethics," *Medical Anthropology Quarterly*, Vol. 6, No. 1, (1992), pp. 49–73.

32. Marshall, p.. 54–55.

33. Beauchamp and Childress, *Principles of Biomedical Ethics*.

34. John F. Burns, "Once Widowed in India, Twice Scorned," *New York Times* (March 29, 1998), p. 1.

3

Respect
for
Tradition

THE standard response of relativists to ethical judgments made by "outsiders" is that "respect for tradition" should render a culture's rituals or customs immune from such criticism. Subcultures in a multicultural society, as well as entire cultures or religions that comprise a majority of a society, understandably seek to preserve their cultural heritage and resist suggestions for change. Tolerance is a virtue, at least according to Western cultural values. Practicing tolerance demands careful scrutiny of alien beliefs and customs before rejecting them out of hand. Yet even on the assumption that a tolerant attitude requires an initial presumption of respect for tradition, how far must it extend? Is the need for tolerance an adequate defense against the legitimacy of making ethical judgments? What if the customs the tradition embodies pose a risk of serious harm or even death to those affected by them? Must we politely refrain from criticism because the Western value that holds tolerance to be a virtue dictates respect for tradition or because our views might be considered unwelcome because they are foreign? Endless paradoxes arise when a Westerner insists on an attitude of tolerance, a value that may itself be alien to another culture. Suppose that culture is intolerant of Western values, such as promoting equality for women and recognizing their reproductive rights. Because tolerance of these Western political values is not part of their repertoire, it seems inconsistent to insist that we maintain tolerance toward their values.

One way of locating the importance of cultural traditions on the moral landscape is to subject particular traditions to the test of fundamental ethical principles. Does the tradition systematically oppress a segment of the population, for example, women, or racial or ethnic minorities? If so, the culture embodies a fundamental injustice. Only if we are prepared to say that oppression of women and minorities is wrong in the Western world but perfectly all right in other societies can we hold a traditional culture immune from criticism. Does the tradition sanction killing, mutilation, or maiming that appears to produce more harm than benefits? If so, we have to see whether those practices can be justified by demonstrating that the harm is outweighed by compensating benefits. Does the tradition involve coercion of individuals either for their own presumed benefit or for the benefit of others? Simply because a custom or ritual is a "tradition" in a culture cannot serve to justify its perpetuation when it quite clearly violates general ethical principles. Principles of justice, nonmaleficence, beneficence, and respect for persons are abstract and difficult to apply, but they can and do serve as a moral yardstick to measure the behavior of individuals and groups.

"Maintain respect for tradition" is a convenient injunction for people in power—usually defenders of the status quo—to keep the system that sustains their power intact. As a practical maxim, "maintain respect for tradition" may well have value for anthropologists conducting fieldwork. Researchers' failure to adhere to the maxim would result in their being expelled from the culture under study or their being denied future access to it. Their role as social scientists is to describe, not to evaluate. But "respect for tradition" cannot serve as an ethical *justification* of an action, custom, or practice. It can only function as an explanation for why people continue to do what they have done for centuries.

This still leaves open the possibility that "respect for tradition" could be justified by an appeal to a fundamental ethical principle if one were found to be applicable. It is possible, for example, that an appeal to the utilitarian principle could serve ultimately to justify the maintenance of some traditions that might at first appear to be harmful. By itself, however, "maintain respect for tradition" cannot provide a moral justification in answer to the question, "How can modern Africans defend a ritual like female genital mutilation?" Female genital mutilation and early marriage are two traditions that have extreme, negative health consequences for girls and women in the parts of the world where these customs persist. A detailed examination of these two traditions may enable us to determine whether they can be ethically justified or merely explained by the factors that sustain them.

Polygyny and Early Marriage

Traditions governing marriage in many countries vary considerably. To take one example, let us consider polygyny (the version of polygamy in which men have more than one wife) and early marriage in Nigeria.[1] The marital practice of polygyny is prevalent among non-Christians in Nigeria as well as in other parts of Africa. It is common among highly educated and prominent people in addition to those who are poorly educated and come from remote parts of the country. Most Africans who practice polygyny are Muslims, and many adhere simultaneously to traditional religions. Nigerian men can have as many as five wives and sometimes more. One Nigerian university professor cited his own polygynous father's remark that "the newest wife is the most loved." Each successive wife tends to be a younger woman, an adolescent, and can even be a girl as young as 8 or 9. Families are often paid a bride price for their female children, and many poor people are eager to have one less mouth to feed in their family. Although the father of the girl may be paid by the husband, it is only a relatively small sum and therefore is not the main factor in the wish of the family to marry off daughters while they are so young.

The practice of early marriage is long-standing in this part of the world. However, some aspects appear to have changed. In earlier times, girls were betrothed at a very young age (often to boys of the same age). When they reached 8 or 9 years of age, they were sent from their parental home to live with the family of their future husband. There they learned the household duties of a wife and mother from the woman (or women) who would become their mother(s)-in-law. A feature of this traditional system, however, was that there was to be no sexual contact between the young girl and her future husband until she reached physical maturity. One writer describes the custom of the Nso' people of the Bamenda Highlands of Kamerun as follows:

> Sometimes a girl was betrothed to a husband as early as when she was still 5 years old. As she grew up, she would spend lengthy periods in the husband's compound or sometimes, in fact, she moved permanently to live in his compound. It was, however, taboo for him to have sexual relations with her before maturity.[2]

This taboo somehow got lost or ceased to be respected, at least in Nigeria, and the 8- or 9-year-old today is expected to have sexual relations as soon as she enters the household of her husband. When she reaches puberty she is at risk of becoming pregnant, with the likely consequences of risks to her health and possibly even to her life.

In the north and also some parts of the east in Nigeria, the people favor child marriage. Key informants told me the situation in rough outline during my visit to Nigeria. In some instances, girls get married at a very young age and then leave their husbands after a month or two. So, by the age of 13, they may have had three or four successive husbands. (No explanation was provided for this pattern.) Girls are typically taken out of school to be put up for marriage. Sometimes the young wives are not permitted to go to a hospital for childbirth even where a health facility exists near her home. The mother-in-law may be opposed to her going to the hospital, saying, "I didn't go to the hospital when I had your husband."

The health consequences for girls and adolescent women put into marriage by their families are disastrous. Because young adolescents are physically immature, they are at high risk once they become pregnant. The stress on their bodies from pregnancy itself carries a risk, but the greatest risk comes with childbirth. Because of their underdeveloped anatomy, many young women experience obstructed labor. According to one authority from Africa, "The medical and social risks of pregnancy are greater for adolescents than for adult women. Rates of prematurity, low-birthweight babies, maternal and infant mortality, anemia, and pre-eclampsia are dramatically higher for adolescent mothers."[3] Most people in Nigerian live in rural areas with no Western-trained doctors and use traditional healers and traditional birth attendants for medical care.

A great many traditional birth attendants are ignorant of human anatomy and hygiene and employ a ritualistic practice known as the *gishiri cut*—a blind incision in the anterior vaginal wall—to enlarge the passage for the emerging infant based on the false belief that obstruction can be remedied in that way. The result in some cases is hemorrhage and death. In a remarkably high proportion of cases this incision cuts into the bladder, resulting in a permanent condition of leaking urine, known as *vesicovaginal fistula*. The woman, often a young adolescent, who leaks urine smells bad, and her husband throws her out of the house. She goes back to the home of her parents, who sometimes accept her but who often also reject her because she smells from leaking urine. Besides, they had already given her out in marriage and did not contemplate having her back. She then turns to the streets and tries to survive by begging and prostitution. Although it is tempting to attribute this grim picture to a shortage of Western trained obstetricians and lack of access of a rural population to hospitals, a deeper explanation is more telling: the traditional practice of early marriage, payment of a bride price, and the cultural prohibition of allowing women to make their own choices about marriage or reproduction.

Many times during my visit to Nigeria I asked: Why do so many Nigerians favor these early marriages? The answer provided by one obstetrician-gynecologist, a Nigerian who treats many of the women suffering from vesico-vaginal fistula, was to safeguard the family's honor. Young marriage is more common among Muslims, who fear that unmarried girls will become promiscuous once they enter adolescence, and as a result the family will be shamed. A daughter's promiscuity brings the family great dishonor, and the family experiences deep shame as a result. There is no worse evil that could befall them than the dishonor of having a promiscuous daughter, one who engages in sex before marriage. Not even the death of the girl as a result of obstructed labor is a worse evil for the family. So, remarked this physician with resignation, this is their scale of values.

This example shows how difficult it is to apply a fundamental ethical principle like beneficence to different cultures. According to a modern, secular scale of values, permanent disability or death of a daughter is considered a far worse consequence for the girl herself and her family than the shame of premarital sex and a resulting pregnancy. For Nigerian Muslims, these values are reversed. It does not seem possible to provide an objective demonstration that early marriage produces a balance of harmful consequences over beneficial ones when members of a culture believe that a daughter's having sex before marriage is a worse evil to the family than that same daughter's death.

Still seeking to understand the cultural values that lead to such unfortunate consequences, I asked the physician who was explaining all this, what is the evidence that girls will actually be promiscuous in this society if they marry later? There is not a great deal of evidence, but apparently there is some. However, the gynecologist remarked, the social practice of early marriage among Nigerian Muslims is not related to the *likelihood* of the occurrence of this undesirable behavior. Given the extremely negative consequence of the shame and dishonor that could result, it is the fear itself that it might happen that drives the behavior. Another explanation offered for the tradition of early marriage is that females in this culture are valued for their reproductive capacity. According to one Nigerian women's health advocate, girls are not educated because their only value is as "vehicles for reproduction."

The Nigerian gynecologist who explained the rationale for early marriage received her professional training in modern scientific medicine. As our conversation ended, she mentioned still other traditional beliefs. Uneducated people, following the lead of traditional birth attendants, adhere to practices from "pagan" religions. The belief system of these religions attributes illness and the possibility of cures to the gods. So, the doctor concluded, if the people do not accept the concept of scientific causality and medical, scientific explanations for the causes and cure of diseases, how can they be expected to take proper preventive steps?

A sobering question. Whose obligation is it, if anyone's, to seek to dispel beliefs that stem from indigenous religions and replace them with beliefs derived from a scientific world view? Would anyone in our own society think it appropriate to try to convince Jehovah's Witnesses of the falsity of their "unscientific" article of faith that they will be denied the opportunity for eternal salvation if they undergo a blood transfusion? It is important for our understanding of cultural and ethical relativism to note that the situation among Nigerians is not a case of Western society seeking to impose cultural beliefs on the native culture. Rather, it is a disparity between educated Nigerians who subscribe to the tenets of modern medicine and Nigerians who live mostly in rural areas and adhere to traditional beliefs and practices.

If polygyny has negative social and health consequences for women, is that a sufficient basis on which to condemn it? Should the custom of placing girls as young as 8 or 9 in marriage—often with a much older man—be condemned on similar grounds? Responses to these questions by those who defend them are instructive.

Defenders of polygyny include some African women who resent the intrusion of Western feminists into a cultural milieu that Africans claim outsiders do not understand and cannot appreciate. Defenders contend that criticism by outsiders of cultural beliefs and practices, such as polygyny and giving 10-year-old girls into marriage, are inherently flawed by the impossibility of adopting a cultural perspective different from one's own. Justifications for such customs can only lie in the traditions and way of life of the culture itself. This is analogous to the cognitive relativism, described in the preceding chapter, to which some anthropologists subscribe.

More pragmatic defenses were offered by a group of physicians, activists, and social scientists who were participants in a workshop that I attended on reproductive health and sexuality. Explanations were offered at two levels: At the societal level, "The society does not see anything wrong in putting 13-year-old girls up for marriage to a 55-year-old man"; and at the individual level, "The 55-year-old man will say, 'This isn't the first time a 13-year-old was put up for marriage and it won't be the last.'" These do serve as explanations, but they could hardly be called ethical justifications. The observation that the society does not see anything wrong with child marriage is the classic relativist position: "Whatever a society approves of is ethically right." The defense that "everyone else is doing it, so why shouldn't I?" is a classic excuse for all sorts of corruption, cheating, and malfeasance everywhere in the world.

A workshop participant mentioned one episode in which women from the North responded to attempts by a Nigerian women's group to bring about reforms intended to benefit women. "Don't do this for us," the women from the North said. "There is nothing wrong with men taking many wives. If my husband didn't have a second wife, I couldn't be here at this conference. Don't try to change the law that allows men to have many wives." This attempt at ethical justification takes the form, "It would be worse for me if polygyny were abolished." This self-interested justification applies to women like the speaker, but not to Nigerian women as a group and surely not to those—presumably unlike herself—who have become sufferers from vesico-vaginal fistula. Moreover, changes in other aspects of the culture might also enable this woman to attend the conference even if she were the sole wife of her husband.

The existence of grassroots women's groups, health advocates of both sexes, and social and legal advocacy organizations in Nigeria clearly show that the traditional culture is undergoing change. If people from within the culture perceive the need for change in some traditional practices to reduce the harms caused by those traditions, it strikes a blow at the major tenet of normative ethical relativism, the view that whatever a culture approves of is ethically right for that culture. As for early marriage among Muslims and ethnic subgroups in the country, which lies at the root of numerous reproductive health problems, that practice is likely to be difficult for Nigerians from other religious or ethnic groups to reform. It is the sort of change that of necessity must come from within the religious or ethnic group in order to gain acceptance by the rural and poorly educated people who suffer most from these practices.

Organizers of the meetings and workshops during my visit to Nigeria invited me to introduce fundamental ethical principles to participants, who would be unfamiliar with bioethics if not also Western philosophical thought. One interdisciplinary group from Ibadan agreed that a strategy for change might be to relate these ethical principles to the culture, the religion, and the existing power relationships. One person said, "The really interesting ethical issue is our own obligation—it's up to us to devise a strategy for change." But another participant ended on a somewhat pessimistic note. She said that "sitting down and talking with these people won't work. You have to use all sorts of methods to bring about change. Methods have to be used to coerce people to do what you want them to do." I did not comment on her proposed method, but found it ironic that in a discussion of ethics this participant appeared to endorse coercion as an appropriate means to achieve the desired end.

Female Genital Mutilation

The ritual known variously as *female circumcision, female genital mutilation,* and *genital surgery* is widely performed in some parts of the world. Female genital mutilation is defended explicitly and implicitly on grounds of "respect for tradition" in the countries where it is practiced. It is carried out on newborns, infants, preadolescents, as a puberty rite, on women just before marriage, on pregnant women, and on women who have just given birth. Just when genital cutting occurs in the life of a girl or woman depends on the region and the traditional or ritual purpose the act is meant to serve. Among the reasons given for this ritual are that it promotes chastity and safeguards virginity, is a religious requirement, fosters group identity, is required for health (prevents maternal and infant mortality) and cleanliness, is aesthetically pleasing and is a prerequisite for women to be marriageable.[4]

Within Egypt, female genital mutilation is performed on girls of different ages, although the typical time is at puberty, and with different degrees of severity (although the most prevalent form is the milder one). It is interesting to note that the relation between female genital mutilation and sexuality also varies in different places where the rite is performed. In Egypt, where sexual relations are prohibited before marriage, the ritual is carried out at puberty. Elsewhere in Africa, however, once having been circumcised in a puberty rite the girl is considered ready to engage in sexual relations.

Estimates range from 85 to 115 million women throughout the world who have been genitally mutilated.[5] This rite is practiced today in 26 African countries, with rates of prevalence ranging from 5% to 99%.[6] One estimate for Nigeria alone puts the prevalence at 50% of all women, totaling more than 30 million.[7] In Somalia the prevalence is estimated to be as high as 98% and in Sudan, 89%. Female genital mutilation is practiced by Muslims, Christians, some animists, and one Ethiopian Jewish sect, but it is not required by any of these religions. Although many people believe it to be a requirement of the Muslim religion, the ritual existed in Africa before Islam entered the continent. Furthermore, neither the Koran nor the sayings of the Prophet Mohammed call for female genital mutilation as a religious requirement.[8]

Female genital mutilation has mild and severe forms. In the "mildest" forms (type I clitoridectomy), a part of the clitoris or the whole organ is removed. In type II clitoridectomy, the entire clitoris and part of the labia minora are removed. The most severe form is total infibulation, in which the clitoris and labia minora are removed and the opening is stitched together to cover the urethra and the entrance to the vagina, leaving a small opening for the passage of urine and menstrual blood. There is also an intermediate form of infibulation that involves less stitching and results in a larger opening. When women have been infibulated, their husbands often have to cut them, usually with a knife, to make sexual intercourse possible on their wedding night. All infibulated women must have the stitching cut to make a large enough opening for childbirth to occur. They are almost always re-infibulated following childbirth, guaranteeing that the trauma will recur at the birth of each child.

Short-term consequences of the procedure include severe pain, infection, trauma, hemorrhage, and even death. If performed in an infant or child and bleeding is prolonged, severe anemia and growth retardation can result. Serious long-term consequences result from infibulation more than from the milder forms of cutting and include formation of cysts and disfiguring scars, abscesses, pain during intercourse, infertility, chronic pain, chronic reproductive and urinary tract infections, obstructed labor, and increased risk of HIV infection. Most (but not all) women permanently lose the ability to achieve sexual pleasure.

Because of these physical complications, which are often accompanied by pain and psychological anxiety and depression, female genital mutilation is viewed by most of the Western world as a significant public health issue. In the United States, Patricia Schroeder, a former member of the House of Representatives from Colorado, argued that when performed on children female genital mutilation should be regarded as a form of child abuse.[9] Representative Schroeder introduced a bill into Congress banning genital cutting, which became a law late in 1996. The International Medical Advisory Panel of the International Planned Parenthood Federation issued a statement declaring that female genital mutilation deserves special consideration as a type of mental and physical abuse of women and children.[10] The American Public Health Association stated that female genital mutilation is a basic violation of human rights and bodily integrity and poses significant health risks.

The people who perform female genital mutilation are primarily traditional birth attendants in most countries. Virtually all are women, and they obviously have a vested interest in continuing the practice as it is a

source of their income and is many times what they could earn as a midwife or healer.[11] However, the picture of legions of ignorant traditional
healers using dirty razors to slice off women's genitals stands in need of
correction. Although this picture is still accurate in many rural communities, there are now medically trained midwives and nurses who carry out
the practice. Medical supplies intended to improve childbirth care are
provided by ministries of health and used by the trained nurses and midwives in the service of their ritual cutting. Despite condemnation by medical associations in most countries, doctors increasingly provide these services. Physicians argue that they can reduce the health risks by using their
skills and antiseptic practices. It is also true that doctors receive a nice additional income from extending their medical services.[12] However, performance of this ritual by a physician does not guarantee safe results. In August 1996 a 14-year-old Egyptian girl bled to death after a doctor did the
cutting. The previous month an 11-year-old Egyptian girl bled to death after the procedure was performed by a barber.[13]

If female genital mutilation is not only physically harmful but also a
violation of a fundamental human right, then it cannot be defended as a
traditional ritual immune to criticism by outsiders to the cultures where it
is practiced. If, on the other hand, as defenders argue, female genital mutilation is accepted and sought by women themselves in the cultures where
it is prominent, then it is arguably not so different from American women
choosing to have breast implants and other forms of cosmetic surgery in
order to appear more feminine.[14] Further complicating the international
picture is that fact that female genital mutilation is used to foment the historical rivalry between the Western, Christian culture and the African and
Arab Muslim civilization.

The cultural practice of female genital mutilation has posed a real
dilemma for those anthropologists who are feminists. On the one hand, as
anthropologists they must maintain a value-free stance in describing and
writing about different cultures. Commitment to the professional ethics of
their field requires them to maintain "respect for the traditions" of the people they study. On the other hand, as feminists, they believe there is something wrong with a practice that not only deprives millions of women of
sexual pleasure, but also produces the well-documented physical harms—

some of them lifelong — in a substantial portion of those women. This is a real dilemma for feminist anthropologists.

Some have recommended an approach that softens the language, in the hopes that it will somehow make the dilemma go away. The authors of one article reject the public health language of "eradication" used by Western opponents who seek to eliminate the practice. The language of eradication is appropriate to germs and infectious diseases, they argue, not to rituals and customs: "It is especially important that we proceed with high regard for the beliefs and concerns of the cultures where it is practiced."[15]

Why do anthropologists urge us to "proceed with high regard for the beliefs and concerns of the cultures that practice female genital mutilation"? Must we proceed with high regard for the beliefs and concerns of the powers in Bosnia who engaged in ethnic cleansing and used a tactic of mass rape of Muslim women in waging their war? Must we hold in high regard the concerns of Tutsis who hacked to death their Hutu neighbors in Rwanda and Burundi? Should we condone infanticide of girl babies in India and China because of the strong cultural preference for sons?

At least three possible explanations exist for the anthropologists' urging. One is the requirement of cultural sensitivity, the need to be aware of cultural differences. A second is the pragmatic reason that criticism from the West will only serve to further entrench traditions in cultures that are skeptical of or even hostile to Western intrusions. The third explanation is the belief that any ethical judgments coming from Western sources constitute cultural imperialism.

These anthropologists state the hope that they can move beyond the impasse of the confrontation between universalism and cultural relativism. Their way of accomplishing this task is to construct an approach respectful of diverse cultural concerns. They reject the phrase *female genital mutilation* in place of the less inflammatory phrase *traditional female surgeries* because "enormous damage can be done by inappropriate choice of language."[16] They avoid talking about rights, noting that some who seek to abolish female circumcision within their own cultures do so by using a framework of women's health rather than women's rights. This may well be a necessary political strategy for bringing about change from within.

But must we conclude that rights language is inappropriate in discussions of the ethics of this ritual?

I believe that this attempt to move beyond the impasse of cultural relativism and universalism does not succeed. It is a valiant attempt, but one that proceeds by emptying cross-cultural judgments of all moral language. Without moral language, ethical judgments cannot exist. The refusal to make ethical judgments means that there is no way to justify efforts to reform social policy or practice. These anthropologists do support such reform, but believe that it can only come from within. In that case, it may be the exercise of political pressure, without accompanying ethical arguments, that might succeed. Just what steps governments or individuals from outside a culture may legitimately take when human rights are violated is a question of international diplomacy and international law. That is quite a different matter from choosing linguistic expressions that embody ethical judgments or those that avoid the language of ethics altogether.

It is curious that the same anthropologists who reject the use of *mutilation* terminology make a linguistic maneuver in the opposite direction that lends a positive connotation to *female circumcision*. They use the term *traditional female surgeries* to describe the procedure. It is true, of course, that the term *mutilation* is not value-neutral; it implies a harsh moral judgment. The difference between mutilation and surgery lies not in a description of the act performed, but in other features that determine what we call the act. When a surgeon cuts off a patient's gangrenous hand to prevent the infection from spreading and killing the patient, we call it *surgical removal of the hand*. When theocratic governments in Muslim countries cut off the hands of people who are charged with stealing, adherents of Islamic law defend it as a legitimate application of retributive justice, whereas non-Islamic critics condemn it as *mutilation*, classifying it as "cruel and unusual punishment."

In adopting the term *surgery* or *operation* for all forms of female circumcision or genital mutilation, anthropologists have chosen what they believe is a value-neutral description, but it is not. Surgery is a practice within a medical or healing tradition, designed to benefit the patient by removing a harmful or potentially dangerous portion of the anatomy. Applied to removal of female genitals, it implies that this ritual practice medically benefits the girl child or woman. But few of the reasons given for this tradition seek to explain or justify it by reference to the health benefits to women. To apply the term surgery to this practice is just as tendentious as to use the word *mutilation*. It implies a healing purpose and connotes the antiseptic practices of the modern, scientific operating theater. Neither the purpose nor the hygienic conditions bear any resemblance to one another.

Most puzzling of all is the anthropologists' attempt to construct an approach "respectful of diverse cultural concerns." The softened language of their policy statement calls for viewing cultural traditions like female genital mutilation "in a new light." These anthropologists end by endorsing and supporting the efforts of individuals and groups *within* countries to abolish the practice, a position inconsistent with their defense of "respect for tradition." Why support those efforts at all? Why not, instead, support the efforts of those who seek to "medicalize" the practice and put it in the hands of skilled physicians who could minimize the trauma, pain, and short- and long-term physical harms to women and thereby continue the tradition?

The anthropologists' carefully worded policy statement urges that the traditional procedures be abandoned in the light of medical information about the damage caused by the practice when performed in the traditional way. But if that is the only reason (dare we add, based on nonmaleficence, the principle of "do no harm"?), an equally sound conclusion would be to urge wider training of physicians and provision of "genital surgeries" in aseptic hospitals. Install a genital surgery ward on the general surgery service. That would be more respectful of cultural concerns, as it would enable the practice of female circumcision to continue but with much reduced morbidity and mortality. This would seem to be the logical conclusion of a position that supports maintaining respect for tradition. The anthropologists are caught in a tug of war between their professional role as anthropologists and their advocacy role as feminists.

Paradoxically, some of the same anthropologists who insist on respect for tradition also speak of "the right to cultural self-determination." There is at least an apparent contradiction in the use of the concept of rights, which many non-Westerners have claimed is a Western concept. Yet anthropologists employ this language in arguments that defend traditional practices against Western critics who say female genital mutilation violates the rights of individuals or the entire class of women. One anthropologist argues that the right to cultural self-determination emerged against "the injustice of colonialism and heavy-handed cultural imperialism" and is therefore a "clearly defensible right."[17] Perhaps so. But then there is the additional problem of potential conflict between the "clearly defensible right" of cultural self-determination and the rights of individual women within those cultures.

If the right of cultural self-determination is a "clearly defensible right," why not also the right of women to be freed from subjection to a cultural ritual perpetuated by centuries of patriarchy in African societies? An anthropologist's refusal to make the moral judgment that female genital mutilation violates women's rights does not rest on a moral defense of genital mutilation. It is, rather, a pragmatic consideration: Female genital mutilation will end only when the practitioners agree that it is the right thing to do. That agreement will not be forthcoming as long as practitioners perceive outsiders as seeking to prescribe their own Western values. A backlash will result against this cultural imperialism, ultimately harming rather than helping the cause of eliminating the traditional practice.

The feminist anthropologist cannot escape between the horns of the dilemma, however valiantly she may try. One author refers to "the unfortunate outcome" of a universalistic pronouncement like "Female circumcision violates women's human rights."[18] Why is that pronouncement "unfortunate"? Because it "sounds like cultural imperialism."[19] The phrase "women's human rights" comes out of North American feminist values and can therefore lead to a backlash against any pronouncement that smacks of Western ethical imperialism.

None of the contentions of anthropologists described so far can compare with the scorn and abuse heaped on a prize-winning essay published in the *Medical Anthropology Quarterly*.[20] The author of the essay apparently had three strikes against him: he was American, living far from the cultures he wrote about; he was male, and these procedures are done on women; and he was a medical student (albeit simultaneously working on a Master's Degree in anthropology). The scathing attack on his essay was mounted in an invited commentary, which was entitled: "Safeguarding Women's Bodies: The White Man's Burden Medicalized."[21] The title itself reveals the animus of the commentary's author, an Egyptian woman and a corresponding editor of the journal. How dare a white, medical man criticize a cultural practice carried out in distant lands on women of color? The commentary finds fault with numerous aspects of the essay, but the focus is a venomous attack on the essay as belonging "to a bygone era of colonial domination" bearing "the characteristic markings of the Western civilization project."[22]

The medical student's essay argues that the anthropological literature has been "inappropriately passive" in response to the international health concerns evident in with female genital mutilation.[23] He characterizes the situation as a dilemma of cross-cultural ethics but comes down on the side of opposing a "practice that is painful, physically disfiguring, medically treacherous, and oppressive to women."[24] He faults his anthropological colleagues for failing to integrate a consideration of the medical complications of female genital mutilation into their writings and says that "the international women's rights movement has not been far off base in considering anthropologists as perpetuating a cover-up."[25]

Upon reading both articles, I can only conclude that the vehemence of the commentator's attack has little to do with the content of the essay and much to do with the essayist's nationality (American), gender (male), chosen profession (medicine), and therefore his lack of qualifications for writing about female genital mutilation in Egypt. It is easy to understand the commentator's defensiveness regarding the essayist's criticism of her colleagues, the value-neutral anthropologists. But mainly she reads the "text" (in preference to the evidence and arguments) of the essay, finding all the earmarks of colonialism in the author's use of language. That language is apparently "coded" in a way that reveals to feminist anthropologists the colonialist underpinnings of people who write about cultures other than their own.

Where does the author of the essay go wrong? For one thing, he refers to the "Western movement of opposition" to female genital mutilation and the "Western influences of industrialization and urbanization" as a force for change. Apparently, use of the word "Western" marks the author as a colonialist. Anyone (especially male) from the West who is presumptuous enough to write about the plight of "the female Other"[26] is immediately a suspect in yet another "Western rescue mission." The commentator rejects the essayist as a neocolonialist who lacks "the minimal requirements for international partnership in feminist struggle."[27]

In a visit I made to Egypt, I was fortunate to escape such attacks. (I was not nearly so fortunate when I wrote an article published in a medical ethics journal in India, as recounted in Chapter 7, or when I delivered a lecture at Wellesley College about son preference in Asia, as noted in the Preface to this book.) I came away from my visit to Cairo with a somewhat different picture from that portrayed in the writings of feminist anthropologists. There I met with Dr. Marie Assaad, who heads the Egyptian female genital mutilation Task Force. She mentioned that one of the participants in the workshop in which we had participated that morning had criticized the term *female genital mutilation*, saying that that language is too harsh and condemnatory. Would it not be better to stick to the term *female circumcision* she asked, but Dr. Assaad defended her use of the stronger term.

Dr. Assaad has been conducting research on female genital mutilation since 1979, long before it attracted attention in the West. She reported the view of physicians who favor providing safer, more skilled procedures by the medical profession. Doctors say, "I can save the life of this girl, and so I am obligated to do that rather than allow her to be placed at risk in the hands of a traditional practitioner." Dr. Assaad is critical of the urgings of these doctors, in part because "saving the lives of young girls" overstates the benefits of having medical practitioners perform the procedure. Another reason for her critical stance is the well-known fact that doctors receive a fee for performing female genital mutilation in their private offices. Even in hospitals, where the practice was legalized for a time by an order from the Minister of Health, the hospital would collect a fee for doing the procedure. During that period of legalization, each hospital established a committee whose task it was to try to discourage the family who brings the girl in for circumcision. Dr. Assaad said that the committee was unlikely to be effective, partly because as an official committee of the hospital it would be eager for the hospital to receive increased revenues. Moreover,

Dr. Assaad noted, once the parents arrive at the hospital with their daughter, they are already resolved to have the girl circumcised.

Until very recently, talking openly about female genital mutilation never occurred in Egypt. This allowed a variety of myths and false beliefs to be perpetuated. For example, women have not typically talked with other women about female genital mutilation, and as a result many circumcised women believe that the practice is universal in Egypt. They cannot believe that some Egyptian women are not circumcised, and they say that women who are not circumcised "would be like men, running around always looking for sex." Dr. Assaad has heard this herself from circumcised women and has replied to them, "I am not circumcised; do you think I am like a man?" A corresponding set of false beliefs has prevailed among the (usually more educated) uncircumcised women in Egypt. They cannot believe that such a large percentage of women are circumcised, and consequently they have not placed this topic on the feminist agenda until recently. I asked whether it is true that men will not consider an uncircumcised girl to be marriageable. She replied that that is not entirely clear. That is the traditional belief, but its truth has not been established by research.

Dr. Assaad contended, along with most critics of the practice, that it is wrong to defend female genital mutilation on the grounds that it is an important tradition within the culture. It is a tradition defended and perpetuated by those who have traditionally held power, and it is practiced in their interests, not in the interests of women, who have not historically been empowered. But she noted that opposition to mobilizing against female genital mutilation has arisen because of attacks on the practice made by American feminists. She confirmed the anthropologists' claim that those attacks have led to a backlash on the part of some Egyptian women, who argue that opposition to the practice must come from within the country.

Analyzing female genital mutilation as the anthropologists have done has not gotten us very far. As one who believes that principles can be used in the service of an ethical analysis, I want next to try that approach. To begin, does female genital mutilation accord with or violate the "respect for persons" principle? The difficulty of applying these general principles is immediately apparent. Infants and young girls cannot consent, dissent, or express any wishes regarding the procedure, so in those cases it is performed nonvoluntarily. Does the principle apply at all to this group? To make the analogy with parental permission to enroll children in research or authorize medical therapy will not do, because those forms of parental authorization are not justified by "respect for persons." Parental authorization for treatment and research maneuvers on children rests on the view that parents are the ones best suited to and most appropriate for protecting this vulnerable population from harm. That justification will not work in the case of female genital mutilation, because parents have their girl children mutilated to protect themselves from shame, not to protect the child from harm.

One uncontroversial conclusion, however, is that it does violate the respect for persons principle when female genital mutilation is performed on girls around the age of puberty, on adolescents, and on women who object or resist. The image of three or four women holding down a screaming, struggling adolescent while the midwife does the cutting is a not-too-subtle portrait of coercion. What can we say about the girls and women who say nothing but passively submit to the ritual? In one interpretation, they are "coerced" by their culture and have no genuine choice. In another interpretation, passive assent still implies voluntariness. However, in cultures in which women have few autonomous choices, where unmarried women are still treated as a possession of their fathers and married women as a possession of their husbands, it is difficult to ascribe genuine autonomy or voluntariness to women generally. The meaning of autonomy as "having a capacity for self-rule" is barely applicable in cultures where women are neither encouraged nor permitted to think and decide for themselves.

There is still a third group: adolescents and women who are eager for the rite to be performed and who look forward to it. Two interpretations exist for this group also. The powerful motivation of wanting to be like one's peers, along with the social significance of rites of passage, can be said to diminish the autonomy of women who are evidently eager to be cut. People with diminished autonomy do not act voluntarily in the full sense. However, this interpretation empties almost all acts of any meaningful component of voluntariness in societies that have a rigid social structure and strong sanctions to comply with norms and traditions. A different interpretation acknowledges that there are, in fact, women who act out of genuine autonomy in wanting their genitals to be cut because they value the norms of desexualization of women and the "bond" female genital mutilation creates with other women in their culture.

The analysis thus far considers "respect for persons" as it applies to individual women undergoing genital mutilation. Applied to the class of women, however, it is easier to conclude that genital mutilation violates this principle. A custom that is aimed at denying women the capacity for sexual pleasure fails to show respect for women as a group. It also fails to show respect for women to mistrust their wish or capacity to remain faithful to their husbands unless their clitoris is excised and their vaginal opening stitched together. The "respect for persons" principle is therefore violated if we consider the effect of the custom on women as a class.

Nonmaleficence is simple to apply, and the conclusion is obvious. Female genital mutilation causes some harm to all its subjects and serious harm to some. It causes pain in all females of whatever age. In many it also causes the array of short-term and long-term harms that have been described. Whether the alleged "benefits" outweigh those harms is to be determined according to the principle of beneficence.

Applying the principle of beneficence raises all the difficulties of the utilitarian calculus: how to predict potential harms and benefits; how to balance physical, health-related harms against the alleged social benefits of female genital mutilation; how to judge the importance of preserving a society's traditional culture in the face of known, predictable harmful consequences, and so on. This would be a much harder balancing act were it not for the strong opposition and efforts at reform made by individual women and women's groups within all of the societies in which female genital mutilation is practiced. If it were solely Western women (and men) who judged the harms of female genital mutilation to outweigh the benefits, the charge of "ethical imperialism" or "neocolonialist judgment" might have merit. But the opposition to this practice and attempts at reform among women in all these cultures—including both women who have themselves been genitally mutilated and those who have not—provides convincing evidence that the unfavorable benefit–risk ratio accorded to female genital mutilation is not solely a product of a Western scheme of values.

An adequate account of the harms and benefits of any medical procedure or cultural practice must begin with solid empirical evidence. There is ample evidence of the harms wrought by female genital mutilation but few data in support of the alleged benefits. Some claims regarding alleged benefits can be readily dismissed as false based on well-confirmed, scientific evidence. The contention that female genitals are unhygienic and "need to be cleaned" is belied by the very consequences of the procedure: If the stitching leaves only a very small opening, urine and menstrual blood collect and cause a foul odor; the creation of a fistula with rectum or bladder causes lifelong incontinence and odor.[28] The falsity of the claim that female genitals will grow to become unwieldy if they are not cut back[29] is demonstrated by the "control group" in nature: all the women in the world who have not been genitally mutilated. Claims regarding the alleged health benefits are also demonstrably false: female genital mutilation does not improve fertility, but does the opposite; nor does it prevent maternal and infant mortality, but again produces the opposite consequences.

As Dr. Marie Assaad and others observe, there is little evidence that avoidance of female genital mutilation will lead to widespread promiscuity, sex before marriage, and pregnancy, the most-feared consequences of failure to circumcise girls. There is also little evidence that uncircumcised women in the cultures where it is practiced behave like men when it comes to sexual behavior. It is true, however, that stitching the vaginal opening will succeed in preserving virginity until marriage. Whether that perceived benefit of female genital mutilation is sufficient to outweigh its myriad harms is a point of contention between defenders and opponents of the practice.

The final alleged benefit—creating a bond among women in the cultures where female genital mutilation is practiced and giving them a sense of belonging—is open to several objections. The data from Assaad's study showed that circumcised women in Egypt falsely believed that all women in that country must be circumcised, and uncircumcised women vastly underestimated the numbers who have been circumcised. The actual fact of having had one's genitals cut had little to do with women's beliefs or their feelings of solidarity. Whatever may be the basis for women's solidarity, it surely does not stem from any communications regarding the facts about genital mutilation.

Moreover, if the international women's movement has shown anything to be true, it is that women from vastly different cultures and racial, religious, and ethnic backgrounds feel a common bond that has nothing to do with the state of their genitalia. The majority of women who attended the International Conference on Population and Development in 1994 in Cairo, and the International Women's Conference the following year in Beijing, were united in their support of women's reproductive rights and their opposition to genital mutilation, and to all forms of oppression against women. The judgment by the feminist anthropologist referred to earlier—that the universalistic pronouncement "female circumcision violates women's human rights" is an "unfortunate outcome"—can only be viewed as an anomaly of anthropologists torn by conflicting ideologies. As anthropologists, they must adhere to the value-neutral ethos of their academic discipline. As feminists, they must stand opposed to traditions that benefit men and harm or oppress women. Ethics supplies us with the principle of beneficence, which can be applied anywhere in the world to people in any situation. The burden of proof lies with those who contend that the benefits of female genital mutilation outweigh the harms it causes.

As for justice, we can only observe that nothing analogous to female genital mutilation is performed on boys and men in these cultures. There is a vocal, worldwide movement opposed to male circumcision, but any resemblance between removal of the male foreskin and virtually all of the forms of female circumcision is remote. There is more than one principle of justice, and for our purposes here we can focus first on distributive justice as an appropriate version for analyzing female genital mutilation. The principle calls for an equitable distribution of society's benefits and burdens. All the burdens fall upon women, as individuals and as a class. Benefits accrue to the traditional circumcisers, the trained midwives and doctors who gain money from performing the ritual.

Are there other beneficiaries? It is probably the case that parents fearful of their daughters' promiscuity if they are not mutilated are greatly comforted by having the ritual carried out. It may also be true that some husbands feel reassured that their infibulated wives will remain faithful to them. What if all these "beneficiaries" of female genital mutilation outnumber the women who suffer the burdens of the ritual? This is one of the classic problems of utilitarianism. One strategy is to contend that the magnitude of pain and suffering of the women is far greater than the comfort or pleasure that accrues to the beneficiaries, regardless of how many individuals are involved. But this strategy has all the drawbacks of assigning utilities to pleasures and pains and has little to do with justice.

Another strategy is to shift from the conception of justice that focuses on distributing benefits and burdens to a different conception, one that takes oppression as its focal point. According to this view, important aspects of oppression are not purely matters of distribution.[30] Some feminists argue that all women are oppressed as a class, not only as individuals, and that this is true in the United States as well as in countries like those where female genital mutilation is practiced.[31] But even those who doubt whether all women everywhere are oppressed cannot but acknowledge that women in traditional, patriarchal societies experience numerous forms of oppression, including being denied an education and any role other than that of wife to a husband and mother to her children. According to this notion of justice, female genital mutilation is only one among many traditional rituals and customs that oppress women and are therefore unjust.

Some have argued that genital mutilation of women should be seen as a human rights violation. If the concept of human rights is meaningful, it follows that we need not hold in high regard cultural beliefs and practices that violate those rights. But the concept of human rights has come under attack too as a peculiarly Western notion that developed out of the historical traditions of Western Europe and North America. We have not yet established whether female genital mutilation should be considered a violation of a fundamental human right. That judgment can be made only after the concept of human rights is elucidated and successfully defended, a task that promises no shortage of conceptual and theoretical problems.

What we can conclude at this point is that even if it succeeds in being a pragmatic maxim for anthropologists, "respect for tradition" is not an ethical principle of any sort, fundamental or derivative. It might be argued that respect for tradition could be considered part of respect for autonomy, but that maneuver will not stand up to ethical scrutiny. Application of the principle "respect for autonomy" cannot require that any actions whatever that flow from the capacity for self-determination must be judged ethically acceptable. People who engage in political torture, commit domestic violence, and sterilize people without their consent may all be acting autonomously, but they do not deserve respect. The same is true for traditions that individuals or a cultural group autonomously accept and adhere to. Some traditional practices are harmful, even evil, some are beneficial, and others are ethically neutral. The mere fact that it is a "tradition" says nothing about the moral value that should be attached to it. Just as laws may be enacted, criticized, or overturned for ethical reasons, so too may customs and traditions be subjected to ethical scrutiny. I have tried to show in the foregoing analysis, using ethical principles, that the traditional practice of female genital mutilation fails in most cases to show respect for persons, produces significant harms and therefore violates nonmaleficence, produces more overall harms than benefits and thus fails to comply with beneficence, and is unjust according to two leading conceptions of justice.

Notes

1. Most of the information in this section was gathered in a visit I made to Nigeria in October 1993 as part of my Ford Foundation project.

2. Godfrey B. Tangwa, "Bioethics: An African Perspective," *Bioethics*, Vol. 10, No. 3 (1996), p. 197.

3. F. T. Sai and K. Newman, "Ethics and Human Values in Family Planning: Africa Regional Perspective," (eds.) Z. Bankowski, J. Barzelatto, and A. M. Capron, *Ethics and Human Values in Family Planning* (COIMS: Geneva, 1989), p. 155.

4. Loretta M. Kopelman, "Female Circumcision/Genital Mutilation and Ethical Relativism," *Second Opinion*, Vol. 20, No. 2 (1994), p. 55; and Nahid

Toubia, *Female Genital Mutilation: A Call for Global Action* (New York: Women, Ink, 1993), p.37.

5. Marion F. MacDorman, "Ban on Female Mutilation/Circumcision," *The Nation's Health*, (Washington, DC: American Public Health Association, September 1996), p. 22.

6. Nahid Toubia, "Female Circumcision as a Public Health Issue," *New England Journal of Medicine*, Vol. 331, No. 11 (1994), p. 712.

7. Nahid Toubia, *A Call*, p. 25.

8. Toubia, *A Call*, p. 31.

9. Patricia Schroeder, "Female Genital Mutilation—A Form of Child Abuse," *New England Journal of Medicine*, Vol. 331, No. 11 (1994), pp. 739–740.

10. International Planned Parenthood Federation, *Statement on Female Genital Mutilation* (November 1991).

11. Toubia, *A Call*, p. 29.

12. Toubia, *A Call*, p. 29.

13. Neil MacFarquhar, "Mutilation of Egyptian Girls: Despite Ban, It Goes On," *New York Times* (August 8, 1996), p. A3.

14. Toubia, *A Call*, p. 35.

15. Sandra D. Lane and Robert A. Rubinstein, "Judging the Other: Responding to Traditional Female Genital Surgeries," *Hastings Center Report*, Vol. 26, No. 3 (1996), p. 38.

16. Lane and Rubinstein, p. 38.

17. Ellen Gruenbaum, "Women's Rights and Cultural Self-Determination in the Female Genital Mutilation Controversy," *Anthropology Newsletter* (May 1995), p. 14.

18. Gruenbaum, p. 14.

19. Gruenbaum, p. 14.

20. Daniel Gordon, "Female Circumcision and Genital Operations in Egypt and the Sudan: A Dilemma for Medical Anthropology," *Medical Anthropology Quarterly*, Vol. 5, No. 1 (1991), pp. 3–14.

21. Soheir Morsy, "Safeguarding Women's Bodies: The White Man's Burden Medicalized," *Medical Anthropological Quarterly*, Vol. 5, No. 1 (1991), pp. 19–23.

22. Morsy, p. 19.

23. Gordon, p. 4.

24. Gordon, p. 12.

25. Gordon, p. 13.

26. Morsy, p. 21.

27. Morsy, p. 22.

28. Gordon, p. 7.

29. Toubia, *A Call*, p. 37.

30. Iris Marion Young, *Justice and the Politics of Difference* (Princeton, NJ: Princeton University Press, 1990).

31. See, for example, Debra DeBruin, "Justice and the Inclusion of Women in Clinical Studies: A Conceptual Framework," (eds.) Anna Mastroianni, Ruth Faden, and Daniel Federman, *Women and Health Research*, Vol. 2 (Washington, DC: National Academy Press, 1994), pp. 127–150; and Susan Sherwin, *No Longer Patient* (Philadelphia: Temple University Press, 1992).

4

The Doctor–Patient Relationship in Different Cultures

WHEN bioethicists from the United States call for recognition of the rights of patients, are they simply expressing their unique American adherence to individualism? The familiar charge of "ethical imperialism" is leveled against proposals that patients in other countries, where individualism is not a prominent value, should nevertheless be granted a similar right to informed consent. While it is true that the doctrine of informed consent focuses on the rights of individual patients, it is not rooted solely in the cultural value of individualism. Rather, it stems from a value many cultures recognize, especially those that aspire to democracy and a just social order: the notion that powerful agents, be they from governmental or nongovernmental organizations, may not invade the personal lives, and especially the bodies, of ordinary citizens.

The prominent American sociologist Renée Fox accurately describes the early focus of American bioethics: "From the outset, the conceptual framework of bioethics has accorded paramount status to the value-complex of individualism, underscoring the principles of individual rights, autonomy, self-determination, and their legal expression in the jurisprudential notion of privacy."[1] Critics of mainstream bioethics within the United States and abroad have complained about the narrow focus on autonomy and the concept of individual rights. Such critics argue that much—if not most—of the world embraces a value system that places the family, the community, or the society as a whole above that of the individual person. But we need to ask: What follows from value systems that accord the individual a lower priority than the group? It hardly follows that individual patients should not be granted a right to full participation in medical decisions. Nor does it follow that individual doctors need not be obligated to disclose information or obtain their patients' voluntary, informed consent. It surely does not follow that the needs of society or the community for organs, bone marrow, or blood should permit those bodily parts or products to be taken from individuals without their permission. What might follow, however, is that patients' families may be fuller participants in decision-making than the patient autonomy model ordinarily requires.

Perhaps we need to be reminded just why American bioethics began with such a vigorous defense of autonomy. It is because patients traditionally had few, if any rights of self-determination: Doctors neither informed patients nor obtained their consent for treatment or for research. In a country founded on conceptions of liberty and freedom, it was at least odd that the self-determination Americans so highly prized in other areas of life was largely absent from the sphere of medical practice. An evolution took place in the United States over a period of many years, from an early court ruling in 1914 that required surgeons to obtain the consent of patients through a series of informed consent cases in the 1950s and 1970s. By the time bioethics became an international field of study, paternalistic medicine had been largely transformed in the United States and patients' rights had been solidly established. The same developments are occurring today in the many developing countries where bioethics has more recently become a topic of interest and study. Although most of these countries lack the tradition of individualism that marks North American culture, the legal guarantee of certain rights of the individual has in the past few decades been one of the goals of social and political reformers.

Cross-cultural misunderstandings can affect the way people in one country perceive a situation in another. Participating in a workshop in the Philippines,[2] I encountered an example of a common cross-cultural misunderstanding about informed consent. The discussion focused on the ethical principle of respect for persons and its role in justifying the need to inform patients and obtain their permission to carry out therapeutic or research procedures. A Filipino physician in the audience objected that informed consent may be needed in the United States, where people do not trust their doctors, but, he said, in the Philippines patients place great trust in their physicians. Doctors do not need to protect themselves against lawsuits by having patients sign a consent form.

Throughout the world (and even at times in the United States), people confuse informed consent with the informed consent document. The Filipino physician misunderstood two things: first, the ethical basis for informed consent; and second, the difference between the *process* of informing and obtaining permission and the piece of paper (the documentation) attesting that the process took place. The ethical judgment that patients should be full participants in their treatment decisions is the ethical justification for the doctrine of informed consent. It is not the protection of the doctor, as the Filipino physician believed, that serves as an ethical basis for the practice. Although it is true that the number of medical malpractice lawsuits in the United States far exceeds that in other countries, especially in the developing world, that phenomenon bears little relation to whether patients lack trust in their doctors.

"Physicians Treat Patients Badly"

"Physicians treat patients badly" was a constant theme in virtually all of the developing countries I visited. Unfortunately, many of the shortcomings in the physician-patient relationship that are all too common in many countries continue to exist in the United States, as well. A major difference is that patients in this country are more aware of their legal and moral rights and are consequently more assertive. An Egyptian physician said that in Egypt there is no process by which consent is obtained in clinical practice. She complained that there is no physician–patient communication, in part because doctors do not have the time. Patients are not told about complications, about medical errors, or anything that transpires in the course of treatment. Patients can get no information whatsoever from doctors about their diagnosis, prognosis, or proposed treatment. Before surgical procedures, papers are signed. But those papers say nothing at all. Patients who ask questions are viewed by the doctors as "impolite," and in any case doctors do not like to answer questions posed by patients.

This Egyptian physician did not seek to defend the customary practices of doctors in her country or to argue that they were reflections of cultural values in Egypt. On the contrary, she was attempting in her work to introduce reforms into medical practice in order to bring about better treatment of patients. When I asked what possible remedies there could be for all these ethical shortcomings, she replied by describing two broad strategies. The first is to document abuses—violations of patients' rights, failures to obtain proper informed consent, and the like; the second is to mount a campaign by lobbying, bringing these issues before the public, and putting cases into court. I asked whether these steps are likely to be effective, and she replied that they can succeed in raising consciousness and awareness and further that people have received some compensation when their cases have reached the courts. Gathering cases and making them public can be used to mount campaigns. By this means reforms might be accomplished. The Egyptian physician's criticism of practices in her own country, and the specific reforms she sought to introduce, show that however different in other ways the culture of Egypt may be from that of Western nations, the ethical ideal that requires physicians to treat their patients with respect is widely acknowledged, if not always honored.

A colleague in Mexico gave a similar account of the lack of recognition of patients' rights in her country.[3] One example was a story told to her by the doorman of her building. His wife was in labor and went to the public hospital. She remained in labor for 2 days, during which time neither the woman nor her husband were told anything about her condition. Eventually she gave birth and was discharged from the hospital while the baby had to remain there for a while longer. Still the couple was told nothing. My colleague expressed her outrage at this situation, blaming the doctors in public hospitals for their unwillingness to disclose information to patients, much less to obtain properly informed consent.

While I agreed that this was an outrage, I noted that things were not so very different years ago in the United States. It is a mere 40 years since the concept of informed consent to treatment was introduced into the legal domain and probably only about 25 years since the practice of obtaining informed consent took root. Still, my Mexican colleague insisted, there are cultural differences. As an example, she cited the pervasive corruption in Latin America as a difference between that region and the North. "What, no corruption in the United States or in Europe?" was my surprised reaction. Of course there is, but we have a much lower tolerance for official corruption, we make strenuous efforts to root it out, and we probably succeed more often in punishing instances that are discovered.

In India I heard more stories about how doctors treat patients badly. One physician described the efforts he and others have been making to inform and enlist the public in opposing unethical medical practices.[4] He recounted a long list of horrors: incompetent doctors practicing poorly or negligently; untrained and unlicensed doctors practicing medicine; physicians overcharging patients; and more. The array of unethical behavior

ranged from genuine malpractice to arrogance and indifference to patients. I asked about legal recourse, and here the situation is just as bleak.
There exists a body called the Medical Council of India, which is supposed to be responsible for monitoring and dealing with the standard of
care delivered by physicians. But this is a peer review system in which doctors protect other doctors. When cases of blatant malpractice are brought
before this council, they fail to find the physician at fault. As a result, nothing is done to remedy instances of actual malpractice or the behavior of incompetent physicians. Patients can, in principle, bring suits against doctors. However, doctors win most of the cases brought to court in spite of
their having committed actual malpractice, and judicial appeals take
many years.

A different group of doctors repeated the same list of horror stories
that I had heard from the first Indian physician, and more. When they
mentioned the "kickback" system, I naively thought they were referring
only to money paid to the referring doctor by the surgeon or specialist to
whom the referral was made. But they meant much more by "kickbacks,"
including demands by the referring doctor that the surgeon perform unnecessary procedures, charge the patient for them, and then give a percentage of the take to the referring doctor. Surgeons and other specialists
who rely on referrals for their practice have to play the game or else they
are not sent a single patient. Thus even doctors who begin by being ethical
and idealistic end up getting caught up in a system in which they must
play or fail to make a living.

All these accounts of bad behavior of physicians toward patients have
little to do with cultural differences or with ethical relativism. They simply
remind us that arrogance, corruption, greed, and indifference are universal character flaws that can be found in human beings throughout the
world, wherever they live and whatever their profession. The chief difference between these countries and the United States lies not in a divergence in the cultural acceptance of such behavior by physicians but,
rather, in the existence of laws and other forms of social control to root out
and punish doctors who violate universally acknowledged ethical norms
and standards of good clinical practice. The efforts of the Egyptian physician and the Indian doctors to bring about reforms in their countries are

evidence of a widespread cross-cultural identification of the same ethical values that ought to govern the doctor–patient relationship everywhere. Respect for persons—in this case, individual patients—was the principle invoked implicitly or explicitly by people from Latin America, Asia, and North Africa in my visits to those regions.

Similarities and Differences

Even in those parts of the world where the cultural traditions differ radically from those in the West, certain values in the doctor–patient relationship are overarching. I participated in a meeting in Nigeria that included several non-English speaking tribal chiefs and native healers. One chief was asked for his views about helping a woman to have an abortion. (Abortion is illegal in Nigeria as in many other countries, but legal prohibitions have never succeeded anywhere in eliminating requests for or performance of the procedure.) Suppose a woman came to him, a traditional healer, asking for an abortion. What would he do? His reply was translated from his native tongue as follows: "If a client comes to me, as a professional, I will help the woman because I have the knowledge to do so." He added, however, that "the community would not be happy."

Here was a medical person—a traditional healer—referring to his "professional" obligation to his patient. He invoked precisely the same consideration most Western physicians would appeal to as a reason why they should help a woman to have an abortion despite the community's disapproval of abortion. Although the cultures may differ in significant ways, the obligations of healers to those who come to them for help remain a cultural universal, one that exists in virtually all societies.

Not every customary practice is properly termed a *tradition*. Values inherent in a social institution such as medical practice may be a reflection of a value in the culture at large, or they may be specific to that particular institution. Lack of recognition and respect for the decision-making autonomy of patients has been a feature of Western medicine throughout most of history and even today remains prominent in other parts of the world. There is a difference, however, between the professional norm in which doctors decide for their patients and a cultural norm that gives family members complete control of another's freedom of decision and action.

Similarly, not every set of norms deserves to be called a *culture*. Although phrases like "the culture of Western medicine" are tossed around, medicine is not a culture in the genuine sense of the term, as anthropologists define it (recounted in Chapter 2). To refer to "the culture of medicine" is to speak metaphorically rather than anthropologically. As one commentator observes: "Used metaphorically, *culture* is everywhere these days. . . . Today the press is full of stories about the 'culture' of the Defense Department, the Central Intelligence Agency . . ., Congress . . ., and any large corporation that happens to be in the news. *GQ* even describes opera as being characterized by 'the culture of booing.'"[5]

Rural areas in many parts of the world still maintain many features of traditional culture in the true sense of the term. Women's health advocates in Mexico reported that in some areas the husband or mother-in-law of a woman decides whether she may visit a physician or whether she may use a method of birth control.[6] This behavior prevails today in rural areas and among indigenous groups and is sanctioned by certain beliefs and values regarding women. For example, women are believed incapable of making their own decisions; or, even if they are capable, they must remain subordinate to men; or the role of women is to reproduce and therefore they should not be permitted to choose to control their own fertility. Control by husbands and mothers-in-law of a woman's fertility is based on the traditional culture and has little to do with the social institution of medicine. Although these sorts of beliefs and values have deep cultural roots they, too, may change over time, as women's health advocates work at the grassroots level and expose women in rural and indigenous communities to the ideas of the global women's movement. Defenders of traditional culture condemn these activists in Mexico and elsewhere as intrusive purveyors of Western feminism who seek to destroy traditional cultural values.

Interestingly, some women's health advocates worry about the effect of introducing values such as autonomy and independence to the women they work with. One social scientist used the example of women with whom they work in a traditional Mexican setting. These women have to ask permission from their mothers-in-law to visit a physician. A mother-in-law may question that decision or refuse to grant permission. The woman then asks the researcher for help. This poses a problem for the researcher: Can the researcher provide some assistance without causing the research subject further psychological damage or harm to her interests? The woman might actually be expelled from her home if the mother-in-law finds out she has gone to a physician without her permission.

While it is no doubt true that some customary practices are rooted in cultural traditions, others may simply have been passed down from one generation to the next as ways of behaving that no one questioned or sought to change. The medical profession has a long history of customary practices, but few qualify as "cultural" traditions. The custom of physicians withholding information from patients and talking, instead, to family members is probably a good example. Everyone from Western anthropologists to physicians in non-Western cultures remark on the difference between the nature of communications between doctors and patients in North America and other parts of the world as if this represents a deep-seated difference in cultural traditions. These commentators probably do not realize, or may have forgotten, that it is only a few decades since physicians in the United States began disclosing diagnoses of fatal illnesses directly to patients. One may call these norms of truth-telling a "tradition," but that would be to distort the more prevalent meaning of "tradition." That meaning is related to the concerns of the ethical relativist—that different societies have distinct and possibly incommensurate ethical values stemming from their cultural diversity.

One commentator suggests that cross-cultural differences in the physician–patient relationship are attributable to different systems of biomedical ethics. Diego Gracia, a professor of public health and history of science in Spain, distinguishes between Mediterranean biomedical ethics and the Anglo-American variety. Gracia notes that patients in Southern European nations are generally less concerned with matters related to informed consent and respect for autonomy than with trust in their physician. Mediterranean bioethics emphasizes virtues rather than rights. Accordingly, the virtue of trustworthiness is more crucial to patients than the right to information.[7]

But Gracia also points to a recent trend in Mediterranean countries, a trend that once again shows the evolution of the physician–patient relationship and the introduction of new ethical values. Gracia notes that in all Mediterranean countries, respect for patients' autonomy and the right of patients to participate in medical decisions have grown extensively in the last decades. Coming some decades after the patients' rights movement began in the United States, this new trend in the Mediterranean countries also includes complaints about health care workers' failure to provide information and for nonconsensual touching.

This phenomenon is one of historical evolution of the doctor–patient relationship rather than a cross-cultural difference between individualistic American culture and the more communitarian or virtue-based value systems in other countries. If the "culture" of medicine has evolved in this way first in the United States and shortly thereafter in some European countries, it is reasonable to suppose that the wider culture—society as a whole—may undergo other changes. No country today is so isolated from the rest of the world that it can remain aloof from and immune to cross-cultural influences.

Conceptions of Autonomy: East and West

A Japanese physician, Noritoshi Tanida, describes sharp differences between features of Japanese and Western culture related to the role of the individual.[8] Tanida says that tradition has left little room for the individual or for individualism in Japan; yet he acknowledges that since the opening of Japan to the West about 130 years ago, Western individualism was introduced into the country. Nevertheless, most Japanese are much less individualistic than are Westerners, a feature that is evident in the decision-making process. In general, Tanida notes, there is no open discussion or clear responsibility, but rather a process of mutual dependency. As a result, the person most affected by a decision may not be informed of what is happening and is not always a part of the decision-making process. The clearest example of this, Tanida holds, is concealing the truth from cancer patients in the practice of clinical medicine.

Another East Asian, Ruiping Fan, puts forth an even stronger view of the difference between East and West with regard to the individual's role in medical decision-making.[9] Fan argues that the Western concept of autonomy, which demands self-determination on the part of the individual, is incommensurable with the East Asian principle of autonomy, which requires family determination. In contending that these two notions of autonomy are incommensurable, Fan insists that there is no shared abstract content between the Western and Eastern principles of autonomy; the two are separate and distinct.

One conclusion that can be drawn from the contrast between East and West is that there simply is no universal ethic regarding disclosure of information, informed consent, and decision-making in medical practice. Not only do these practices differ as a matter of fact in different societies, but they are incompatible. This conclusion is obviously true for the descriptive thesis of ethical relativism: Truth-telling, informed consent, and decision-making about medical treatment vary in different cultures. Furthermore, if we accept Fan's account, a conceptual variation exists as well; autonomy means something different in East Asia from what it signifies in the West.

The East Asian principle of autonomy holds that "Every agent should be able to make his or her decisions and actions harmoniously in cooperation with other relevant persons."[10] Thus when patients and family are in harmony, they decide together. That situation probably prevails most of the time in Western medical practice as well. However, it is the family who has the final authority to make clinical decisions in accordance with the East Asian principle. According to Ruiping Fan, if a patient requests or refuses a treatment while a relevant family member disagrees with that decision, the doctor should not simply follow the patient's wish but should urge the patient and the family to negotiate and come to an agreement before the physician will act. It is the family that constitutes the autonomous social unit, and the physician may not act contrary to their decision.

This example of cultural diversity raises the enduring question of normative ethical relativism: Has Western bioethics arrived at the ethically right position with regard to respecting the individual autonomy of the patient? Is the practice in other cultures of deferring to the patient's family, or leaving the decision in the hands of the physician, right in those cultures although it would be wrong in the United States?

The emphasis on autonomy, at least in the early days of bioethics in the United States, was never intended to cut patients off from their families by insisting on an obsessive focus on the patient. Rather, it was intended to counteract the predominant mode of paternalism on the part of the medical profession. In fact, there was little discussion of where the family entered in and no presumption that a family-centered approach to sick patients was somehow a violation of the patient's autonomy. Most patients want and need the support of their families whether or not they seek to be autonomous agents regarding their own care. Respect for autonomy is perfectly consistent with recognition of the important role that families play when a loved one is ill. Autonomy has fallen into such disfavor among some ethicists in the United States that the pendulum has begun to swing in the direction of families, with urgings to "take families seriously"[11] and even to consider the interests of family members equal to those of the competent patient.[12]

Fan says that some people may deny that what he refers to as the "East Asian principle of autonomy" can even be characterized as a principle of autonomy. He nevertheless defends his use of the term, noting that the word for autonomy in the Chinese language is often used not only for individuals, but also for units like a family or a community. The same is true in the English language: In its political sense, *autonomy* means "self-rule" and can therefore apply to communities, countries, and, as in Mexico, universities.

Fan demonstrates that the East Asian principle of autonomy has significant implications for truth-telling, informed consent, and advance directives in the East Asian clinical setting. If a physician directly informs a patient about a diagnosis of a terminal disease instead of first telling a member of the family, that would be extremely rude and inappropriate. Interestingly, however, while East Asian custom allows the family to choose a treatment on behalf of a competent patient, the family may not readily refuse a treatment on behalf of a competent patient. This is evidently because of the underlying assumption that a treatment recommended by a physician will be beneficial to the patient, whereas it is at least questionable whether a withholding or withdrawing of treatment is in the interests of a competent patient.

So when it comes to actually making medical decisions, who should decide? Should it be patients themselves in the West, in accordance with the principle of autonomy as "self-determination," and families of patients in the East, in accordance with the "family-determination–oriented" principle? There is little doubt at this point that in the United States the patient with decisional capacity holds the moral and legal right to decide, with very rare exceptions. Those exceptions include some cases in which a pregnant woman's refusal of an intervention is deemed harmful to the life or health of the fetus (forced cesarean sections are the clearest example of this) and the situation in which physicians judge a treatment to be "medically futile" and take the decision-making out of the patient's hands. But these exceptions are contested by those who contend that pregnant women should have all the rights of other competent patients and that a physician's assessment that a treatment is "medically futile" should not replace the patient's wish for the treatment, which may have psychological value.

So we are left with ethical relativism. As Ruiping Fan puts it: "Which principle is more true: the Western principle of autonomy or the East Asian principle of autonomy? Who should give up their own principle and turn to the principle held by the other side?"[13] Fan's own solution is to adopt the procedural principle of freedom, allowing both Western and East Asian people to follow their respective and incommensurable principles of autonomy. Interestingly, Fan's solution appeals to a higher principle, that of freedom or liberty. He acknowledges as much and articulates the principle of freedom commonly associated with Western philosophical and political thought: "Every group of people as well as every single individual has freedom to act as they see appropriate, insofar as their action does not harm other people."[14] That sounds remarkably like something John Stuart Mill might have written.

Application of this principle appears to grant to an individual patient the right to reject the cultural custom of family autonomy in favor of individual decision-making. But would it really? If East Asian patients insisted on their freedom to act as they deem appropriate, doing so might damage family harmony, so perhaps other people would be harmed after all. Ruiping Fan does not raise the explicit question of what individual patients or physicians might do, but refers only to "Western and East Asian people" being free to follow their respective principles of autonomy. It leaves ambiguous the status of the individual patient in East Asia and possibly also the role of a family in the West that seeks to follow the family-determination notion of autonomy.

Is this a relativist solution? Fan says no, it is not to surrender to ethical relativism, "but to secure the most reasonable in a peaceful way in this pluralist world."[15] This reply embraces tolerance and is a practical accommodation to cross-cultural diversity. If not a surrender to relativism, how can we characterize Fan's position? Fan himself describes this type of thought as a "transcendental argument for a content-less principle that ought to be employed in a secular pluralist society."[16] This merely replaces the puzzling with the obscure. Philosophy should seek to explain and clarify, not to obfuscate and muddy. We have to do better.

Truth-Telling

In the Western world the custom of withholding information from patients goes back at least as far as Hippocrates. Hippocrates admonished physicians to perform their duties

> calmly and adroitly, concealing most things from the patient while you are attending to him. Give necessary orders with cheerfulness and sincerity, turning his attention away from what is being done to him; sometimes reprove sharply and emphatically, and sometimes comfort with solicitude and attention, revealing nothing of the patient's future or present condition.[17]

Does this ancient practice represent a tradition of some cultural group? If so, which one? Ancient Greek tradition, carried down through the Greco-Roman empire? That would not have been a likely influence on Asian medical practice. If it is part of any "culture" at all, it is that of the medical profession (speaking metaphorically), renowned throughout the ages for its paternalism. Medical paternalism remains the rule rather than the exception in Asian and Latin America, and it persists to a somewhat lesser extent in some parts of Western Europe, as well.

The shift in attitude toward disclosing the diagnosis to cancer patients began to occur in the United States in the late 1960s, a millennial moment since the time of Hippocrates. Although often portrayed as a cultural tradition, one in which many countries diverge from the preeminence accorded to the individual in the United States, nondisclosure by physicians to patients appears rather to have been a nearly universal customary practice dictated by medical professionals throughout the world.

But things change. Attitudes and practices of physicians in the United States have undergone a striking reversal in the past three decades. A study conducted in 1961 revealed that 90% of physicians did not inform their patients of the diagnosis of cancer.[18] When that study was redone in 1977, it revealed that 98% of doctors usually informed patients of the diagnosis of cancer.[19] It is entirely possible that such changes will begin to occur in other countries as well. Evidence suggests that this has already begun to happen.

These changes do not require us to impugn the motives of physicians who have thought it best not to tell patients they have cancer, nor is it to condemn the benevolence that undergirds medical paternalism in general. Now, as in the past, most justifications for withholding information from patients have rested implicitly or explicitly on an appeal to the principle of beneficence. If the behavior of doctors in the United States has changed in the past three decades or so, it is not because the principle of beneficence no longer serves as a justification or that physicians no longer act from benevolent motives. It is simply that the competing ethical principle of respect for autonomy has taken priority over the principle of beneficence in motivating and justifying physicians' behavior. Once it became evident that patients wished to know their diagnoses (or already knew they had cancer in spite of families and physicians conspiring to keep the news from them), and once physicians came to realize that disclosing a diagnosis of cancer did not typically cast the patient into a deep depression and very rarely, if ever, led to documented cases of patients committing suicide, then benevolent paternalism could no longer be sustained on ethical grounds.

From the earliest moments of modern bioethics, some people worried about the alleged requirement always to "tell the truth." In response to the claim that patients have "a right to know" their diagnosis and prognosis, challengers replied: what about "the right *not* to know?" Of course, there is no inconsistency here. People have a right to receive information, if they want it, and also the right to refuse to receive that information. That is precisely what "respect for persons" supports: respect for the wishes and values of the individual patient.

This is the point at which the philosophical distinction between ultimate moral principles and specific rules of conduct becomes critical. "Respect for persons" is a fundamental, or ultimate, ethical principle. The imperative "tell patients the truth about their condition" is a specific rule of conduct. Moreover, respecting a particular patient's wish not to know is perfectly consistent with the general obligation to disclose to patients their diagnosis. This also demonstrates the distinction between ethical universals and moral absolutes. "Always tell patients the truth about their condition" would be the moral absolute in this case, clearly a different imperative from one that mandates respect for the wishes of patients.

On this analysis, the answer to the question of how the case of truth telling to patients fits into the debates over ethical relativism is simple (relatively speaking). No universal ethical mandate exists to tell patients the truth about their terminal illness. Nor is it the case that telling the patients the truth is right in some countries or cultures and wrong in others. Moreover, to contend that the principle of autonomy mandates disclosure misinterprets how that ethical principle should be applied. Respect for autonomy means, among other things, acting in a way that respects the values of individuals. Individuals' values often mirror the predominant values of their country or culture, but they do not always do so. When they do, we must be sensitive to those values and respectful of the people who hold them.

A lingering problem, however, is that doctors often do not know or do not take the time or trouble to find out the patient's values. They take the family's word for whether the patient "can handle" the information. Or they simply honor the family's wish not to tell the patient. Here is where the practice in the United States is most likely to diverge from that in other

countries. Because respect for the patient's autonomy has become entrenched in American medical practice, most physicians will probably not
automatically comply with the family's wish not to reveal a diagnosis of
cancer or other fatal or terminal illness.

It is clear from published reports in the medical and bioethical literature that doctors in other countries do readily honor a family's request not
to tell the patient a diagnosis of cancer or other terminal illness. I believe
that behavior is as much a reflection of the still dominant paternalism of
physicians as it is an expression of a cultural value. When respect for autonomy is not recognized as an ethical principle in medical practice,
physicians see no need to find out whether a patient wants to know the diagnosis of cancer or terminal illness. Medicine has always been paternalistic and hierarchical. In some ways, the culture of medicine remains paternalistic in the United States, as anyone can attest who has heard physicians
urge the omission of "scary" items from consent forms.

A medical oncologist from Italy, who had practiced for a while in the
United States, reported what she had learned in medical school.[20] The
Italian Deontology Code, written by the Italian Medical Association, included the following statement: "A serious or lethal prognosis can be hid-
den from the patient, but not from the family."[21] That was in the late
1970s. The Deontology Code was revised in 1989, with this statement:
"The physician has the duty to provide the patient—according to his cultural level and abilities to understand—the most serene information about
the diagnosis, the prognosis and the therapeutic perspectives and their
consequences. . . . Each question asked by the patient has to be accepted and answered clearly." The code goes on to grant to physicians the
well-known "therapeutic privilege" of withholding information if disclosure would be harmful to the patient, and in that case the information
must be communicated to the family. But the revised code still represents
a sharp reversal from the presumption of nondisclosure in the code of a
mere decade earlier.

The Italian oncologist who wrote about this shift stated her belief that
ethics is connected to cultural values and varies in different societies. She
rejected a belief in "absolute values" in favor of respecting the pluralism of
different cultures. This was by way of background to her contention that

"the Italian society is not prepared for the American way." She explained further, saying that even today Italians believe that patients will never acquire enough knowledge to enable them to understand what physicians tell them and therefore to participate in their own care. Italians still believe that protecting an ill family member from painful information prevents the sick person from suffering alone, from isolation, and is essential for keeping the family together.

Is it reasonable to expect that these attitudes will gradually be transformed, just as similar attitudes were in the United States several decades ago? The Italian oncologist waffled a bit on this point. On the one hand, she stated her belief that "Italians should not borrow the American way." On the other hand, she urged Italians to learn from Americans and "try to find a better Italian way." As examples of changes taking place within the medical profession, she noted courses in bioethics in universities and medical meetings on truth telling and communicating with patients. In the end, she reached the conclusion that "the only way to respect both Italian ethical principles and the patient's autonomy and dignity is to let the patient know that there are no barriers to communication and to the truth."[22] What is most peculiar is the reference to "Italian ethical principles." Withholding information from patients is not a function of ethnic traditions but rather of how the medical profession has historically conducted its practice in most places in the world. It is also a class phenomenon, since doctors are typically better educated than most of their patients and question the ability of patients to fully understand what they have been told.

A mere 5 years after its 1989 revision, the Italian code of medical ethics was revised once again. The revision reflected the "constantly changing relationship between the medical profession and society, and between physicians and patients."[23] In the newly revised code, the "Italian way" has come very close to the "American way." Article three of the new code adds to the physician's obligation expressed in the 1989 code "to respect the dignity of the human being" the additional obligation to respect the patient's freedom of choice. Article four of the new code adds the physician's obligation to respect the rights of the individual, and extensive revisions of the doctrine of informed consent are in conformity with other modern codes of ethics. The code mandates respect for the decisional autonomy of the patient, even in cases in which the life of the patient is threatened.[24]

Equally striking are revisions on the topic of confidentiality. Whereas the earlier Italian code permitted doctors to conceal the truth from the patient and disclose it to the next of kin, the new code essentially prohibits nondisclosure to the patient and disclosure to a third party. Two exceptions to this rule are, first, when the patient specifically authorizes disclosure to others and, second, when there is potential for harm to a third party.[25] It would be absurd to conclude that "Italian ethical principles" have changed in this brief interlude between the 1989 code and the more recent revisions. Instead, as the authors of an article describing the new code observe, "from a paternalistic attitude in which the physician, for the good of the patient, felt authorised and justified to set aside the personal requests of the patient and even to violate his wishes, a therapeutic alliance has evolved, in which the two partners together try to decide on the clinical choices that best promote the patient's wellbeing."[26]

Changes are also occurring in Asia, a region of the world often cited as adhering to family and group values almost to the exclusion of recognizing the importance of the individual. A Japanese physician observes that the concept of informed consent has recently been recognized in his country, yet he acknowledges that most Japanese physicians withhold information about diagnosis and prognosis from their patients who have cancer.[27] It is reasonable to wonder whether "informed consent" means the same thing in Japan as it does in the West. One report notes that the Bioethics Council of the Japanese Medical Association introduced the idea of "Japanese informed consent," which was to be carried out in accordance with the prevailing medical paternalism in that country.[28] A survey in Japan showed that 67% of physicians would disclose the diagnosis to patients with early cancer, but only 16% would tell those with advanced cancer. Studies from other countries show that many patients do want to be informed of a diagnosis of cancer, but a discrepancy exists between patients' preferences and physicians' attitudes.[29]

A physician speaking at an international conference about truth-telling in Japanese medicine[30] described a number of cultural features that help to explain physicians' reluctance to disclose a bad prognosis. That reluctance stems from patients' unwillingness to receive such information, which in turn is based on deeper cultural roots. Patients want to have an "edited" version of the truth. They enter a tacit conspiracy with their family and the physician to avoid a difficult subject. This results in the family taking over all responsibility and decisions for the patient's illness. Although many patients will guess and come to know the truth eventually, they still will not ask directly. This behavior is rooted in the Japanese ethos in which silent endurance is a virtue. The aim is to make dying easier, not to invoke a dogma of telling patients the truth. Patients want to die as calmly and peacefully as possible, and that goal is more readily achieved if they remain ignorant of their prognosis. Relatives assume the burden of making an intuitive judgment of whether the patient wants to know the diagnosis and can handle it. Not to accept one's death gallantly is worse than death itself. Physicians, patients, and families all want to avoid a "disgraceful upset" that conveying bad new could produce. The physician who explained all this echoed what others discussing medicine in Japan have said: Despite powerful influences from Western countries, Japan is not totally Westernized, yet the Japanese do not want to stick to their old traditions completely. The physician ended by saying that the Japanese people must achieve a new type of death education, with more ethical emphasis, closer to the Western style of dealing with death.

But let us assume that a cultural gap does exist between North American practices of disclosing bad news to patients and different customs in other parts of the world. What should we conclude about whether one cultural practice is "right" and the other "wrong"? How does this example fit into the debates over ethical relativism?

The answer depends entirely on how the question is framed and how the situation is described. Consider the following alternative descriptions.

1. Doctors and patients in the United States believe that patients should be told the truth about a diagnosis of terminal illness. Doctors and patients in other countries believe that doctors should tell the family but not the patient. The ethical principle of "respect for autonomy" mandates that doctors treat patients as autonomous individuals and so must inform them about their illness. The truth-telling practice in the United States

conforms to this principle and is ethically right, whereas the nondisclosure practice in other countries violates this practice and is ethically wrong.

2. Autonomy is the predominant value in North American culture. Doctors and patients in the United States adhere to an autonomy model of disclosure in medical practice. Family-centered values are more prominent than individual autonomy in other cultures. Doctors and patients in these cultures adhere to a family-centered practice of disclosure of terminal illness. Therefore, it is right to disclose to a patient a diagnosis of terminal cancer in the United States and wrong to make that same disclosure in the other countries.

3. Autonomy is the predominant value in North American culture, but disclosure of terminal illness by doctors to patients is nevertheless a fairly recent practice. The U.S. population comprises many recent immigrants, and some cultural groups adhere to family-centered values from their country of origin, especially in specific matters such as disclosure of terminal illness. Family-centered values predominate in other countries, but practices such as disclosure of a diagnosis of terminal illness have begun to change in those places. "Respect for persons" requires that in any country or culture, doctors should discuss with their patients whether they want to receive information and make decisions about their medical care or whether they want the physician to discuss these matters only with the family.

The third description is obviously the "right" answer. What is wrong with the other two descriptions shows what is frequently amiss in debates over ethical relativism. Description 1 has two main flaws. The first is the common failing of distorting or misusing the principle of respect for autonomy. The principle does not require inflicting unwanted information on people; rather, it requires first finding out how much and what kind of information they want to know and then respecting that expressed wish. When the principle of autonomy is interpreted in that way, nothing automatically follows regarding whether patients should be told the truth about their diagnosis. The second flaw is the assumption that all people in a country or culture have the same attitudes and beliefs toward the values that predominate in that culture. In a Los Angeles study of senior citizens' attitudes toward disclosure of terminal illness, in no ethnic group did

100% of its members favor disclosure or nondisclosure to the patient. Forty-seven percent of Korean-Americans believed that a patient with metastatic cancer should be told the truth about the diagnosis, 65% of Mexican-Americans held that belief, 87% of European-Americans believed patients should be told the truth, and 89% of African-Americans held that belief. If physicians automatically withheld the diagnosis from Korean-Americans because the majority of people in that ethnic group did not want to be told, they would be making a mistake almost 50% of the time.[31]

Description 2 is flawed for one of the same reasons that description 1 is flawed: It presupposes that all people in a country or culture have the same attitudes and beliefs toward the values that predominate in that culture. That assumption is clearly false, as the Los Angeles study just cited demonstrates. In a multicultural society such as the United States, ethical relativism poses an array of problems not likely to arise in countries that enjoy a common cultural heritage (if any such countries still remain). "Multiculturalism is good," its proponents contend.[32] Whether or not that is true, it surely causes difficulties for doctors and patients.

Notes

1. Renée C. Fox, "The Evolution of American Bioethics: A Sociological Perspective," (ed.) George Weisz, *Social Science Perspectives on Medical Ethics* (Philadelphia: University of Pennsylvania Press, 1990), p. 206.

2. The workshop, part of my Ford Foundation project, took place in Davao, Mindanao, in December 1995.

3. This interview took place in February 1996 during my second Ford Foundation project.

4. This interview took place in April 1994 in Bombay.

5. Christopher Clausen, "Welcome to Postculturalism," *The Key Reporter*, Vol. 62, No. 1 (1996), p. 2.

6. This meeting took place during my Ford Foundation visit to Mexico in February 1993.

7. Diego Gracia, "The Intellectual Basis of Bioethics in Southern European Countries," *Bioethics*, Vol. 7, No. 2/3 (1993), pp. 100–101.

8. Noritoshi Tanida, "Bioethics Is Subordinate to Morality in Japan," *Bioethics*, Vol. 10 (1996), pp. 202–211.

9. Ruiping Fan, "Self-Determination vs. Family-Determination: Two Incommensurable Principles of Autonomy," *Bioethics*, Vol. 11 (1997), pp. 309–322.

10. Fan, p. 316.

11. James Lindemann Nelson, "Taking Families Seriously," *Hastings Center Report*, Vol. 22 (1992), pp. 6–12.

12. John Hardwig, "What About the Family?" *Hastings Center Report*, Vol. 20 (1990), pp. 5–10.

13. Fan, p. 322.

14. Fan, p. 322.

15. Fan, p. 322.

16. Fan quotes this phrase from H. Tristram Engelhardt, Jr., *The Foundations of Bioethics*, 2nd edition (New York: Oxford University Press, 1996).

17. Citation from President's Commission for the Study of Ethical Problems in Medicine and Biomedical and Behavioral Research, *Making Health Care Decisions* (Washington, DC: Government Printing Office, 1982), Vol. 1, p. 32.

18. D. Oken, "What To Tell Cancer Patients: A Study of Medical Attitudes," *Journal of the American Medical Association*, Vol. 175 (1961), pp. 1120–1128.

19. Dennis H. Novack, Robin Plumer, Raymond L. Smith, Herbert Ochitill, Gary R. Morrow, and John M. Bennett, "Changes in Physicians' Attitudes Toward Telling the Cancer Patient," *Journal of the American Medical Association*, Vol. 341 (1979), pp. 897–900.

20. Antonella Surbone, "Truth-Telling to the Patient," *Journal of the American Medical Association*, Vol. 268 (1992), pp. 1661–1662.

21. Surbone, p. 1661.

22. Surbone, p. 1662.

23. Vittorio Fineschi, Emanuela Turillazzi, and Cecilia Cateni, "The New Italian Code of Medical Ethics," *Journal of Medical Ethics*, Vol. 23 (1997), p. 238.

24. Fineschi, Turillazzi, and Cateni, pp. 241–242.

25. Fineschi, Turillazzi, and Cateni, p. 243.

26. Fineschi, Turillazzi, and Cateni, p. 241.

27. Atsushi Asai, "Should Physicians Tell Patients the Truth?" *Western Journal of Medicine*, Vol. 163 (1995), pp. 36–39.

28. Tanida, p. 208.

29. Asai, p. 36.

30. Shin Ohara, "Truth-Telling and We-Consciousness in Japan: Some Biomedical Reflections on Japanese Civil Religion," unpublished paper presented at the conference, "Ethics Codes in Medicine and Biotechnology," Freiburg, Germany, October 12–15, 1997.

31. Leslie J. Blackhall, Sheila T. Murphy, Gelya Frank, Vicki Michel, and Stanley Azen, "Ethnicity and Attitudes Toward Patient Autonomy," *Journal of the American Medical Association*, Vol. 274, No. 10 (1995), pp. 820–825.

32. Blaine J. Fowers and Frank C. Richardson, "Why Is Multiculturalism Good?" *American Psychologist*, Vol. 51, No. 6 (1996), pp. 609–621.

5

Relativism
and
Multiculturalism

CROSS-CULTURAL judgments not only traverse national boundaries from one part of the globe to another. They also occur within any nation that is multicultural, especially in a country like the United States, which experiences continual waves of immigration from all regions of the world. Cultural pluralism poses a challenge to physicians and patients alike in the multicultural United States, where immigrants from many nations and diverse religious groups visit the same hospitals and doctors as does the mainstream, autonomy-minded majority population.

Multiculturalism is defined as "a social–intellectual movement that promotes the value of diversity as a core principle and insists that all cultural groups be treated with respect and as equals."[1] This sounds like a value that few enlightened people could find fault with, but it produces dilemmas and leads to results that are, at the least, problematic if not counterintuitive.

The predominant norm in the United States of disclosing to the patient a diagnosis of serious illness is not universally accepted even among long-standing citizens comprising ethnic or religious subcultures. Moreover, "respect for autonomy" as an ethical principle continues to be misunderstood and perhaps even deliberately misrepresented. The following episode is illustrative.

An orthodox rabbi was invited to deliver a lecture on Jewish medical ethics at a medical school. The rabbi outlined some of the leading precepts of Jewish medical ethics and sought to compare them with their counterparts in contemporary secular bioethics. Understandably, given his commitment to Orthodox Judaism, he undertook to defend the precepts of Jewish medical ethics in those instances where they conflict with the secular version. The rabbi told the story of a man with an abiding fear of cancer who visited his doctor because he was worried about a small growth on his upper lip. The pair had a long-standing physician–patient relationship, and the doctor was aware of the patient's deep fear of cancer. When the patient paid a return visit following a delay in which the biopsy was examined, he said to the doctor: "It isn't cancer, is it?" The physician, after a brief hesitation, reassured the patient that he did not have cancer.

The rabbi commended the physician's action, saying that secular bioethics would insist on patient autonomy and require that the doctor tell the truth, thereby instilling great anxiety in the patient. The rabbi went on to say that Jewish medical ethics does not place autonomy above all other values, noting that respect for autonomy has little place in Jewish medical ethics. Instead, the physician, as the person with medical expertise, has the obligation to do whatever is best for the patient, based on that expertise, and the patient—a layperson—does not have "a right to know" everything the doctor may discover. The impression the rabbi sought to convey was that secular bioethics mandates truth-telling to patients even when it means inflicting unwanted information. The more benevolent Jewish medical ethics allows for withholding diagnostic information and can support telling "white lies" to avoid harming the patient.

I am not concerned here to debate the general merits of the contemporary practice of disclosing a diagnosis of cancer. Nor do I intend to argue that a value placed on truth-telling should prevail universally, inside medical practice as well as in the world at large. But I did object, when I listened to the rabbi's lecture, to his omission of a few critical pieces of information. He had taken the story of the patient fearful of cancer from an article in a medical journal written by the physician, who also was a protagonist in the story. In the published article, the physician explained his action and sought to justify it, not by defending the tradition of medical paternalism but with a different rationale.

The physician believed he had an obligation to be truthful to his patients. He normally does disclose a diagnosis of cancer. However, reflecting in this case on the patient's extreme and irrational fear, the physician reasoned as follows. Although the patient did, indeed, have a form of cancer, it was a tiny growth confined to a small region of the skin, of a type that does not spread and could not have metastasized. The growth could be completely removed and there would be no further consequences. What this patient thought of as cancer—what he feared so deeply—was not the condition he actually had. So, the doctor reasoned, he could be conveying as much of an untruth by telling this man he had cancer, given the patient's conception of that disease. Telling the patient he did not have cancer was the doctor's way of saying that the man did not have what he most feared—a fatal illness, and that was being truthful.

One might quibble with the semantics of this little story: Did the doctor lie or not? Was it not literally a lie? Or was the "larger" truth the physician intended to convey the "real" truth? Is it correct to say that the doctor was being truthful, even though he did not literally "tell the truth"? However those philosophical questions may be answered, the lessons that flow from the tale are several. The first lesson highlights the difference between an absolutist ethics and a universalist ethics. An absolutist ethics contains exceptionless rules: "Never lie. Never break promises. Always tell the truth." Few people anywhere (rigid Kantians excepted) defend this form of absolutism. Every ethical rule has some exceptions, which can be justified in the usual manner by appealing to higher principles that would be violated if one adhered to the rule.

A universalist ethics, on the other hand, maintains that fundamental ethical principles exist and can be used to justify specific rules. This brings us to the second lesson of the story: The fundamental principle that underlay the physician's response to the patient was the "respect for persons" principle. The rabbi who recounted the story sought to demonstrate the superiority of Jewish medical ethics because the beneficence of the physician's white lie was ethically defensible—and so it was.

Where the rabbi erred, however, was in his contention that secular medical ethics, with its reigning principle of "respect for autonomy," would require inflicting on the patient the unwanted information that he had cancer. The principle of "respect for persons" is broader than the principle of "autonomy," although the latter concept is often the relevant interpretation of what follows from "respect for persons." In this episode, the concept of autonomy played a different role from what usually follows from "respect for persons." This was a matter of the physician revealing to the patient the nature of his ailment and describing it to him in a way that the patient would properly understand. In recognizing and being sensitive to the patient's fear of cancer, the physician showed respect for the patient's beliefs and values. The physician reasoned that this patient would misunderstand a diagnosis of cancer. Neither respect for persons nor beneficence mandates providing information that a patient would not fully comprehend.

The third lesson from this story is a reminder that the much-maligned principles of bioethics are often misused or abused by people conducting an ethical analysis. I neither know nor care whether the rabbi was intentionally distorting the application of the principle "respect for autonomy" to demonstrate the beneficent nature of Jewish medical ethics. It was simply a mistake to say that the principle of autonomy as employed in secular bioethics requires that doctors always "tell the truth" to patients, even when it may cause terrible harm.

A circumstance that arises frequently in a multicultural urban setting like New York City is one that medical students bring to ethics teaching conferences. The patient and family are recent immigrants from a culture in which the patient is normally not told a diagnosis of cancer, but, rather, physicians inform the family. The medical students wonder whether they are obligated to follow the family's wish, thereby respecting their cultural custom, or whether to abide by the ethical requirement at least to explore with patients their desire to receive information and to be a participant in their medical care. When medical students presented such a case in one of the conferences I co-direct with a physician, the dilemma was heightened by the demographic picture of the medical students themselves. Among the 14 students, 11 different countries of origin were represented. Those students had come to the United States themselves to study, or their parents had immigrated from countries in Asia, Latin America, Europe, and the Middle East.

The students began their comments with remarks like, "where I come from, doctors never tell the patient a diagnosis of cancer" or "in my country, the doctor always asks the patient's family and abides by their wishes." The discussion centered on the question whether the physician's obligation is to act in accordance with what contemporary medical ethics dictates in the United States or to respect the cultural difference of their patients and act according to the family's wishes. Not surprisingly, the medical students were divided on the answer to this question.

Medical students and residents are understandably confused about their obligation to disclose information to a patient when the patient comes from a culture in which telling a patient she has cancer is rare or unheard of. They ask, "Should I adhere to the American custom of disclosure or the Argentine custom of withholding the diagnosis?" That question is miscast because there are some South Americans who want to know if they have cancer and some North Americans who do not. It is not, therefore, the cultural tradition that should determine whether disclosure to a patient is ethically appropriate, but rather the patient's wish to communicate directly with the physician, to leave communications to the family, or something in between. It would be a simplistic, if not unethical, response on the part of doctors to reason that "This is the United States, we adhere to the tradition of patient autonomy, therefore I must disclose to this immigrant from the Dominican Republic that he has cancer."

Most patients in the United States do want to know their diagnosis and prognosis, and it has been amply demonstrated that they can emotionally and psychologically handle a diagnosis of cancer. The same may not be true for recent immigrants from other countries, and it may be manifestly untrue in certain cultures. Although this, too, may change in time, several studies point to a cross-cultural difference in beliefs and practice regarding disclosure of diagnosis and informed consent to treatment.

One study was mentioned in the preceding chapter: a survey that examined differences in the attitudes of elderly subjects from different ethnic groups toward disclosure of the diagnosis and prognosis of a terminal illness and regarding decisionmaking at the end of life.[2] This study found marked differences in attitudes between Korean-Americans and Mexican-Americans, on the one hand, and African-Americans and European-Americans, on the other. The Korean-Americans and Mexican-Americans were less likely than the other two groups to believe that patients should be told of a prognosis of terminal illness and also less likely to believe that the patient should make decisions about the use of life-support technology. Both the Korean- and Mexican-Americans surveyed were more likely to have a family-centered attitude toward these matters; they believed that the family and not the patient should be told the truth about the patient's diagnosis and prognosis. The authors of the study cite data from other countries that bear out a similar gap between the predominant "autonomy model" in the United States and the family-centered model prevalent in European countries as well as Asia and Africa.

The study cited was conducted at 31 senior citizen centers in Los Angeles. It is worth noting that the people surveyed were all 65 years old or older. Not surprisingly, these senior citizens had values closer to the cultures of their origin than the African-Americans and European-Americans who were born in the United States. Another unsurprising finding was that among the Korean-American and Mexican-American groups, older subjects and those with lower socioeconomic status tended to be opposed to truth-telling and patient decision-making more strongly than the younger, wealthier, and more highly educated members of the same groups. The authors of the study draw the conclusion that physicians should ask patients if they want to receive information and make decisions regarding treatment or whether they prefer that their families handle such matters.

Far from being at odds with the "autonomy model," this conclusion supports it. To ask patients how much they wish to be involved in decision-making does show respect for their autonomy: Patients can then make the autonomous choice about who should be the recipient of information or the decision maker about their illness. What would fail to show respect for autonomy is for physicians to make these decisions without consulting the patient at all. If doctors spoke only to the families but not to the elderly Korean-American or Mexican-American patients without first approaching the patients to ascertain their wishes, they would be acting in the paternalistic manner of the past in America and in accordance with the way many physicians continue to act in other parts of the world today. Furthermore, as noted in the preceding chapter, if physicians automatically withheld the diagnosis from Korean-Americans because the majority of people in that ethnic group did not want to be told, they would be making an assumption that would result in a mistake almost 50% of the time.

Intolerance and Overtolerance

A medical resident in a New York hospital questioned a patient's ability to understand the medical treatment he had proposed and doubted whether the patient could grant truly informed consent. The patient, an immigrant from the Caribbean islands, believed in voodoo and sought to employ voodoo rituals in addition to the medical treatment she was receiving. "How can anyone who believes in that stuff be competent to consent to the treatment we offer?" the resident mused. The medical resident was an observant Jew who did not work, drive a car, or handle money on the sabbath and adhered to Kosher dietary laws. Both the Caribbean patient and the Orthodox Jew were devout believers in their respective faiths and practiced the accepted rituals of their religions.

The patient's voodoo rituals were not harmful to herself or to others. If the resident had tried to bypass or override the patient's decision regarding treatment, the case would have posed an ethical problem requiring resolution. Intolerance of another's religious or traditional practices that pose no threat of harm is, at least, discourteous and at worst, a prejudicial attitude. It also fails to show respect for persons and their diverse religious and cultural practices. But it does not (yet) involve a failure to respect persons at a more fundamental level, which would occur if the doctor were to deny the patient her right to exercise her autonomy in the consent procedures.

At times, however, it is the family that interferes with the patient's autonomous decisions. Two brothers of a Haitian immigrant were conducting a conventional Catholic prayer vigil for their dying brother at his hospital bedside. The patient, suffering from terminal cancer and in extreme pain, had initially been given the pain medication he requested. Sometime later a nurse came in and found the patient alert, awake, and in excruciating pain from being undermedicated. When questioned, another nurse who had been responsible for the patient's care said that she had not continued to administer the pain medication because the patient's brothers had forbidden her to do so. Under the influence of the heavy dose of pain medication, the patient had become delirious and mumbled incoherently. The brothers took this as an indication that evil spirits had entered the patient's body and, according to the voodoo religion of their native culture, unless the spirit was exorcised it would stay with the family forever, and the entire family would suffer bad consequences. The patient manifested the signs of delirium only when he was on the medication, so the brothers asked the nurse to withhold the pain medication, which they believed was responsible for the entry of the evil spirit. The nurse sincerely believed that respect for the family's religion required her to comply with the patient's brothers' request, even if it contradicted the patient's own expressed wish. The person in charge of pain management called an ethics consultation, and the clinical ethicist said that the brothers' request, even if based on their traditional religious beliefs, could not override the patient's own request for pain medication that would relieve his suffering.

There are rarely good grounds for failing to respect the wishes of people based on their traditional religious or cultural beliefs, but when beliefs issue in actions that cause harm to others, attempts to prevent those harmful consequences are justifiable. An example that raises public health concerns is a ritual practiced among adherents of the religion known as Santería, people from Puerto Rico and other groups of Caribbean origin. The ritual involves scattering mercury around the household to ward off bad spirits. Mercury is a highly toxic substance that can harm adults and causes grave harm to children. Shops called *botánicas* sell mercury as well as herbs and other potions to Caribbean immigrants who use them in their healing rituals. According to one study in New York City, 44% of the Caribbean people and 27% of the Latin American people in the survey said they used mercury or carried it on their person.

Some immigrants from the West Indies and Latin America believe that mercury can attract good things quickly. Believers use a few drops to clean their floors or mix it with bathwater or perfume. Some even swallow the mercury to cure indigestion or wear it around their neck as a good-luck charm. In a survey of 41 botánicas in New York City, nearly 93% sold one to four capsules of mercury daily. Physicians worried about the health effects, particularly on small children, and planned a study to test hundreds of children in the South Bronx for mercury poisoning. One toxicologist remarked on the problem of freedom of religion, saying that "it's a social and cultural issue."[3]

The public health rationale that justifies placing limitations on people's behavior to protect others from harm can justify prohibiting the sale of mercury and enforcing penalties for its domestic use for ritual purposes. Yet the Caribbean immigrants could object: "You are interfering with our religious practices, based on your form of scientific medicine. This is our form of religious healing and you have no right to interfere with our beliefs and practices." It would not convince this group if a doctor or public health official were to reply: "But ours is a well-confirmed, scientific practice while yours is but an ignorant, unscientific ritual." It may very well appear to the Caribbean group as an act of cultural imperialism: "These American doctors with their Anglo brand of medicine are trying to impose it on us."

Belief System of a Subculture

Some widely held ethical practices have been transformed into law, such as disclosure of risks during an informed consent discussion and offering to patients the opportunity to make advanced directives in the form of a living will or appointing a health care agent. Yet these can pose problems for adherents of traditional cultural beliefs. In the traditional culture of Navajo Native-Americans, a deeply rooted cultural belief underlies a wish not to convey or receive negative information. A study conducted on a Navajo Indian reservation in Arizona demonstrated how Western biomedical and ethical concepts and principles can come into conflict with traditional Navajo values and ways of thinking.[4] In March 1992, the Indian Health Service adopted the requirements of the Patient Self-Determination Act, but the Indian Health Service policy also contains the following proviso: "Tribal customs and traditional beliefs that relate to death and dying will be respected to the extent possible when providing information to patients on these issues."[5]

The relevant Navajo belief in this context is the idea that thought and language have the power to shape reality and to control events. The central concern posed by discussions about future contingencies is that traditional beliefs require people to "think and speak in a positive way." When doctors disclose risks of a treatment in an informed consent discussion, they speak "in a negative way," thereby violating the Navajo prohibition. The traditional Navajo belief is that health is maintained and restored through positive ritual language. This presumably militates against disclosing risks of treatment as well as avoiding mention of future illness or incapacitation in a discussion about advanced care planning. Western-trained doctors working with the traditional Navajo population are thus caught in a dilemma. Should they adhere to the ethical and legal standards pertaining to informed consent now in force in the rest of the United States and risk harming their patients by "talking in a negative way"? Or should they adhere to the Navajo belief system with the aim of avoiding harm to the patients but at the same time violating the ethical requirement of disclosure to patients of potential risks and future contingencies?

The authors of the published study draw several conclusions. One is that hospital policies complying with the Patient Self-Determination Act are ethically troublesome for the traditional Navajo patients. Because physicians who work with that population must decide how to act, this problem requires a solution. A second conclusion is that "the concepts and principles of Western bioethics are not universally held."[6] This comes as no surprise. It is a restatement of the thesis of descriptive ethical relativism. The question for normative ethics remains: What follows from these particular facts of cultural relativity? A third conclusion the authors draw, in light of their findings, is that health care providers and institutions caring for Navajo patients should reevaluate their policies and procedures regarding advanced care planning.

This situation is not difficult to resolve, ethically or practically. The Patient Self-Determination Act does not mandate that patients actually make an advance directive; it requires only that health care institutions provide information to patients and give them the opportunity to make a living will or appoint a health care agent. A physician or nurse working for the Indian Health Service could easily fulfill this requirement by asking Navajo patients if they wish to discuss their future care or options without introducing any of the negative thinking. The authors of the published study acknowledge one of its limitations: The findings reflect a more traditional perspective, and the full range of Navajo views is not represented. Thus it is possible that some patients who use the Indian Health Service may be willing or even eager to have frank discussions about risks of treatment and future possibilities, even negative ones.

It is more difficult, however, to justify withholding from patients the risks of proposed treatment in an informed consent discussion. The article about the Navajo beliefs recounts an episode told by a Navajo woman who is also a nurse. Her father was a candidate for bypass surgery. When the surgeon informed the patient of the risks of surgery, including the possibility that he might not wake up, the elderly Navajo man refused the surgery altogether. If the patient did, indeed, require the surgery and refused because he believed that telling him of the risk of not waking up would bring about that result, then it would be justifiable to withhold that risk of surgery. Should not that possibility be routinely withheld from all patients, then, because the prospect of not waking up could lead other people— Navajos and non-Navajos alike—to refuse the surgery? The answer is no, but it requires further analysis.

Respect for autonomy grants patients who have been properly informed the right to refuse a proposed medical treatment. An honest and appropriate disclosure of the purpose, procedures, risks, benefits, and available alternatives, provided in terms the patient can understand, puts the ultimate decision in the hands of the patient. This is the ethical standard according to Western bioethics. A clear exception exists in the case of patients who lack decisional capacity altogether, and debate continues regarding the ethics of paternalistically overriding the refusal of marginally competent patients. This picture relies on a key feature that is lacking in the Navajo case: a certain metaphysical account of the way the world works. Western doctors and their patients generally do not believe that talking about risks of harm will produce those harms (although there have been accounts that document the "dark side" of the placebo effect). It is not really the Navajo values that create the cross-cultural problem, but rather their metaphysical belief system holding that thought and language have the power to shape reality and control events. In fact, the Navajo values are virtually identical to the standard Western ones: fear of death and avoidance of harmful side effects. To understand the relationship between cultural variation and ethical relativism, it is essential to distinguish between cultural variations that stem from a difference in values and ones that can be traced to an underlying metaphysics or epistemology.

Recall the Chilean woman in an earlier chapter who defended the action of the indigenous people engaged in ritual killing of their infants and then blamed the government for banning the practice. The indigenous group said that a drought ensued because they were unable to appease the Gods with their ritual sacrifice. The woman who told the story rebuked me for appealing to "scientific" beliefs about the cause of droughts, saying "that's merely a belief, just different from the tribe's belief." If tolerance of other cultures requires a suspension of trust in the scientific method for drawing factual conclusions, then many people in most parts of the world are guilty of intolerance. We need not abandon our beliefs about causal efficacy in physics or biology in an attempt to determine what follows from the facts of cultural relativity.

Against this background, only two choices are apparent: insist on disclosing to Navajo patients the risks of treatment and thereby inflict unwanted negative thoughts on them; or withhold information about the risks and state only the anticipated benefits of the proposed treatment. Between those two choices, there is no contest. The second is clearly ethically preferable. It is true that withholding information about the risks of treatment or potential adverse events in the future radically changes what is required by the doctrine of informed consent. It essentially removes the "informed" aspect, while leaving in place the notion that the patient should decide. The physician will still provide some information to the Navajo patient, but only the type of information that is acceptable to the Navajos who adhere to this particular belief system. True, withholding certain information that would typically be disclosed to patients departs from the ethical ideal of informed consent, but it does so to achieve the ethically appropriate goal of beneficence in the care of patients.

The principle of beneficence supports the withholding of information about risks of treatment from Navajos who hold the traditional belief system, but so, too, does the principle of respect for autonomy. Navajos holding traditional beliefs can act autonomously only when they are not thinking in a negative way. If doctors tell them about bad contingencies, that will lead to negative thinking, which in their view will fail to maintain and restore health. The value of both doctor and patient is to maintain and restore health. A change in the procedures regarding the informed consent discussion is justifiable based on a distinctive background condition: the Navajo belief system about the causal efficacy of thinking and talking in a certain way. The less-than-ideal version of informed consent does constitute a "lower" standard than that which is usually appropriate in today's medical practice, but the use of a "lower" standard is justified by the background assumption that that is what the Navajo patient prefers.

What is relative and what is nonrelative in this situation? There is a clear divergence between the Navajo belief system and Western science. That divergence leads to a difference between what sort of discussion is appropriate for traditional Navajos in the medical setting and what is standard in Western medical practice. According to one description, "always disclose the risks as well as the benefits of treatment to patients," the conclusion points to ethical relativism. A more general description, one that heeds today's call for cultural awareness and sensitivity, would be: "carry out an informed consent discussion in a manner appropriate to the patient's beliefs and understanding." That obligation is framed in a nonrelative way. A heart surgeon would describe the procedures, risks, and benefits of bypass surgery in one way to a patient who is another physician, in a different way to a mathematician ignorant of medical science, in yet another way to a skilled craftsman with an eighth grade education, and still differently to a traditional Navajo. The ethical principle is the same; the procedures differ.

Obligations of Physicians

The problem for physicians is how to respond when an immigrant to the United States acts according to the cultural values of her native country, values that differ widely from accepted practices in American medicine. Suppose an African immigrant asks an obstetrician to perform genital surgery on her baby girl. Or imagine that a Laotian immigrant from the Iu Mien culture brings her 4-month-old baby to the pediatrician for a routine visit and the doctor discovers burns on the baby's stomach. The African mother seeks to comply with the tradition in her native country, Somalia, where the vast majority of women have had clitoridectomies. The Iu Mien woman admits that she has used a traditional folk remedy to treat what she suspected was her infant's case of a rare folk illness.

What is the obligation of physicians in the United States when they encounter patients in such situations? At one extreme is the reply that in the United States physicians are obligated to follow the ethical and cultural practices accepted here and have no obligation to comply with patients' requests that embody entirely different cultural values. At the other extreme is the view that cultural sensitivity requires physicians to adhere to the traditional beliefs and practices of patients who have emigrated from other cultures.

A growing concern on the part of doctors and public health officials is the increasing number of requests for genital cutting and defense of the practice by immigrants to the United States and European countries. Although it has been illegal in the United States since 1997, evidence has come to light that requests are being made and honored to do the procedure. Secretary of Health and Human Services Donna Shalala said in early 1998: "It's illegal, it's inhumane and we've got to be clear about that. At the same time, we have to be culturally sensitive in explaining to those immigrants who might put their girls at risk that the practice has harmful physical and psychological consequences."[7]

A Somalian immigrant living in Houston said he believed his Muslim faith required him to have his daughters undergo the procedure; he also stated his belief that it would preserve their virginity. He was quoted as saying, "It's my responsibility. If I don't do it, I will have failed my children."[8] Another African immigrant living in Houston sought a milder form of the cutting she had undergone for her daughter. The woman said she believed it was necessary so her daughter would not run off with boys and have babies before marriage. She was disappointed that Medicaid would not cover the procedure and planned to go to Africa to have the procedure done there. A New York City physician was asked by a father for a referral to a doctor who would do the procedure on his 3-year-old daughter. When the physician told him this was not done in America, the man accused the doctor of not understanding what he wanted.[9]

However, others in our multicultural society consider it a requirement of "cultural sensitivity" to accommodate in some way to such requests of African immigrants. Harborview Medical Center in Seattle sought just such a solution. A group of doctors agreed to consider making a ritual nick in the fold of skin that covers the clitoris, but without removing any tissue. However, the hospital later abandoned the plan after being flooded with letters, postcards, and telephone calls in protest.[10]

A physician who conducted research with East African women living in Seattle held the same view as the doctors who sought a culturally sensitive solution. In a talk she gave at my medical school department, she argued that Western physicians must curb their tendency to judge cultural practices different from their own as "rational" or "irrational." Ritual genital cutting is an "inalienable" part of some cultures, and it does a disservice to people from those cultures to view it as a human rights violation. She pointed out that in the countries where female genital mutilation is practiced, circumcised women are "normal." Like the anthropologists who argue for a "softer" linguistic approach, this researcher preferred the terminology of "circumcision" to that of "female genital mutilation."

One can understand and even have some sympathy for the women who believe they must adhere to a cultural ritual even when they no longer live in the society where it is widely practiced. But it does not follow that the ritual is an "inalienable" part of that culture, because every culture undergoes changes over time. Furthermore, to contend that in the countries where female genital mutilation is practiced, circumcised women are "normal" is like saying that malaria or malnutrition is "normal" in parts of Africa. That a human condition is statistically normal implies nothing whatever about whether an obligation exists to seek to alter the statistical norm for the betterment of those who are affected.

Some Africans living in the United States have said they are offended that Congress passed a law prohibiting female genital mutilation that appears to be directed specifically at Africans. France has also passed legislation, but its law relies on general statutes that prohibit violence against children.[11] In a recent landmark case, a French court sent a Gambian woman to jail for having had the genitals of her two baby daughters mutilated by a midwife. French doctors report an increasing number of cases of infants who are brought to clinics hemorrhaging or with severe infections.

Views on what is the appropriate response to requests to health professionals for advice or referrals regarding the genital mutilation of their daughters vary considerably. Three commentators gave their opinions on a case vignette in which several African families living in a U.S. city planned to have the ritual performed on their daughters. If the procedure could not be done in the United States, the families planned to have it done in Africa. One of the parents sought advice from a health professional.

One commentator, a child psychiatrist, commented that professional ethical practice requires her to respect and try to understand the cultural and religious practices of this group.[12] She then cited another ethical requirement of clinical practice: her need to promote the physical and psychological well-being of the child and refusal to condone parenting practices that constitute child abuse according to the social values and laws of her city and country.[13] Most of what this child psychiatrist would do with the mother who comes to her involves discussion, mutual understanding, education, and the warning that in this location performing the genital cutting ritual would probably be considered child abuse.

The psychiatrist would remain available for a continuing dialogue with the woman and others in her community, but would stop short of making a child abuse report because the woman was apparently only considering carrying out the ritual. However, the psychiatrist would make the report if she had knowledge that the mother was actually planning to carry out the ritual or if it had already been performed. She would make the child abuse report reluctantly, however, and only if she believed the child to be at risk and if there were no other option. She concluded by observing that the mother is attempting to act in the best interest of her child and does not intend to harm her.[14] The psychiatrist's analysis demonstrates the possible ambiguities of the concept of child abuse. Is abuse determined solely by the intention of the adult? Should child abuse be judged by the harmful consequences to the child, regardless of the adult's intention? Of course, if a law defines the performance of female genital mutilation as child abuse, then it is child abuse, from a legal point of view, and physicians are obligated to report any case for which there is a reasonable suspicion.

The second commentator, a clinical psychologist and licensed sex therapist, would do many of the same things as the child psychiatrist, but would go a bit further in finding others from the woman's community and possibly another support network.[15] Like most other commentators on female genital mutilation, this discussant remarked that "agents of change must come from within a culture."[16]

The third commentator on this case vignette was the most reluctant to be critical. A British historian and barrister, he began with the observation that "a people's culture demands the highest respect."[17] On the one hand, he noted that custom, tradition, and religion are not easily uprooted. On the other hand, he pointed out that no human practice is beyond questioning.[18] He contended that the debate over the nature and impact of female circumcision is a "genuine debate," and the ritual probably had practical utility when it was introduced into the societies that still engage in it. Of the three commentators, he voiced the strongest opposition to invoking the child abuse laws because it "would be an unwarranted criminalization of parents grappling in good faith with a practice that is legal and customary in their home country."[19] In the end, this discussant would approach the parents "much as a lawyer would address a jury," leaving the parents (like a jury) to deliberate and come to an informed decision. He would also involve the girls in this process because they are adolescents and should have input into the deliberations.

It is tempting to wonder whether the involvement of adolescent girls in deliberations of their parents would, in traditional Gambian culture, be even remotely considered, much less accepted. The "lawyer–jury–adolescent involvement" solution looks to be very Western. If these families living in the United States still wish to adhere to their cultural tradition of genital mutilation, is it likely that they will appreciate the reasoned, deliberative approach this last commentator proposed?

Exactly where to draw the line in such cases is a difficult matter to determine. Presumably, one could go further than any of these commentators and inform the African families that because U.S. law prohibits female genital mutilation, which has been likened to child abuse, a health professional would be obligated to inform relevant authorities of an intention to commit child abuse. Conceivably, U.S. authorities could prevent immigrants from returning to this country if they have gone to Africa to have a procedure performed that would be illegal if done within the United States. But this is a matter of law, not ethics, and would involve a gross invasion of privacy because, to enforce the ruling, it would be necessary to examine the genitals of the adolescent girls when these families sought reentry into the United States. That would be going much too far and would deserve condemnation as "ethical imperialism." Because the cutting would already have been done, punitive action toward the family could not succeed in preventing the harm.

Another case vignette was presented in a different article describing a Laotian woman from the Mien culture who immigrated to the United States and married a Mien man. When she visited her child's pediatrician for a routine 4-month immunization, the doctor was horrified to see five red and blistered quarter-inch-round markings on the child's abdomen.[20] The mother explained that she used a traditional Mien "cure" for pain because she thought the infant was experiencing a rare folk illness among Mien babies characterized by incessant crying and loss of appetite, in addition to other symptoms. The "cure" involves dipping a reed in pork fat, lighting the reed, and passing the burning substance over the skin, raising a blister that "pops like popcorn." The popping indicates that the illness is not related to spiritual causes; if no blisters appear, then a shaman may have to be summoned to conduct a spiritual ritual for a cure. As many as 11 burns might be needed before the end of the "treatment." The burns are then covered with a mentholated cream.

The Mien woman told the pediatrician that infection is rare and the burns heal in a week or so. Scars sometimes remain but are not considered disfiguring. She also told the doctor that the procedure must be done by someone skilled in burning because if a burn is placed too near the line between the baby's mouth and navel, the baby could become mute or even retarded. The mother considered the cure to have been successful in the case of her baby because the child had stopped crying and regained her appetite. Strangely enough, the pediatrician did not say anything to the mother about her practice of burning the baby, no doubt from the need to show "cultural sensitivity." She did, however, wonder later whether she should have said something because she thought the practice was dangerous and also cruel to babies.

One commentator on this case proposed using "an ethnographic approach" to ethics in the cross-cultural setting.[21] This approach need not result in a strict ethical relativism, however, because one can be respectful of cultural differences and at the same time acknowledge that there are limits. What is critical is the perceived degree of harm; some cultural practices may constitute atrocities and violations of fundamental human rights. The commentator argued that the pediatrician must first seek to understand the Mien woman in the context of her world before trying to educate her in the ways of Western medicine. The commentator stopped short of providing a solution, but noted that many possible resolutions can be found for cross-cultural ethical conflicts. Be that as it may, we still need to determine which of the pediatrician's obligations should take precedence: to seek to protect her infant patient (and possibly also the Mien woman's other children) from harmful rituals or to exhibit cultural sensitivity and refrain from attempts at re-education or critical admonitions.

A second pair of commentators assumed the anthropologists' non-judgmental stance. These commentators urged respect for cultural diversity and defended the Mien woman's belief system as entirely rational: "It is well grounded in her culture; it is practiced widely; the reasons for it are widely understood among the Iu Mien; the procedure, from a Mien point of view, works."[22] This is a culturally relative view of rationality. The same argument could just as well be used to justify female genital mutilation. Nevertheless, the commentators rejected what they said was the worst choice: simply to tolerate the practice as a primitive cultural artifact and do nothing more. They also rejected the opposite extreme: a referral of child abuse to the appropriate authorities. The mother's actions did not constitute intentional abuse, because she actually believed she was help-ing the child by providing a traditional remedy. Here I think the commen-tators are correct, especially because making a formal charge of child abuse can have serious consequences that could ultimately run counter to the best interests of the child.

What did these commentators recommend? Not to try to prohibit the practice directly, which could alienate the parent. Instead, the pediatrician could discuss the risk of infection and suggest safer pain remedies. The doctor should also learn more about the rationale for and technique of the traditional burning "cure." The most she should do, according to these commentators, is consider sharing her concerns with the local Mien com-munity, not with the mother alone.

There is in these commentaries a great reluctance to criticize, scold, or take legal action against parents from other cultures who employ painful and potentially harmful rituals that have no scientific basis. This attitude of tolerance is appropriate against the background knowledge that the parents do not intend to harm the child and are simply using a folk remedy widely accepted in their own culture. But what puzzles me is the idea that "cultural sensitivity" must extend so far as to refrain from providing a solid education to these parents about the potential harms and the infliction of gratuitous pain. In a variety of other contexts, we accept the role of physicians as educator of patients. Doctors are supposed to tell their patients not to smoke, to lose weight, and to have appropriate preventive medical check-ups such as Pap smears, mammograms, and proctoscopic examinations.

Pediatricians are thought to have an even more significant obligation to educate the parents of their vulnerable patients: inform them of steps that minimize the risks of sudden infant death syndrome, tell them what is appropriate for an infant's or child's diet, and give them a wide array of other social and psychological information designed to keep a child healthy and flourishing. Are these educational obligations of pediatricians appropriate only for patients whose background culture is that of the United States or Western Europe? Should a pediatrician not attempt to educate parents who, in their practice of the Santería religion, sprinkle mercury around the house? The obligation of pediatricians to educate and even to urge parents to adopt practices likely to contribute to the good health and well-being of their children, and to avoid practices that will definitely or probably cause harm and suffering, should know no cultural boundaries.

My position is consistent with the realization that Western medicine does not have all the answers. This position also recognizes that some traditional healing practices are not only not harmful but may be as beneficial as those of Western medicine. The injunction to "respect cultural diversity" could rest on the premise that Western medicine sometimes causes harm without compensating benefits (which is true) or on the equally true premise that traditional practices such as acupuncture and herbal remedies, once scorned by mainstream Western medicine, have come to be accepted side by side with the precepts of scientific medicine. Typically, however, respect for multicultural diversity goes well beyond these reasonable views and requires toleration of manifestly painful or harmful procedures such as the burning remedy employed in the Mien culture. We ought to be able to respect cultural diversity without having to accept every single feature embedded in traditional beliefs and rituals.

The reluctance to impose modern medicine on immigrants from a fear that it constitutes yet another instance of "cultural imperialism" is

misplaced. Is it not possible to accept non-Western cultural practices side
by side with Western ones, yet condemn those that are manifestly harmful
and have no compensating benefit except for the cultural belief that they
are beneficial? The commentators who urged respect for the Mien
woman's burning treatment on the grounds that it is practiced widely, the
reasons for it are widely understood among the Mien, and the procedure
works, from a Mien point of view, seemed to be placing that practice on a
par with practices that "work" from the point of view of Western medicine.
Recall that if the skin does not blister, the Mien belief holds that the illness may be related to spiritual causes and a shaman might have to be
called. Should the pediatrician stand by and do nothing if the child has a
fever of 104° F and the parent calls a shaman because the skin did not blister? Recall also that the Mien woman told the pediatrician that if the burns
are not done in the right place, the baby could become mute or even retarded. Must we reject the beliefs of Western medicine regarding causality
and grant equal status to the Mien beliefs? To refrain from seeking to educate such parents and even to exhort them to alter their traditional practices is unjust, as it exposes the immigrant children to health risks that are
not borne by children from the majority culture.

It is heresy in today's postmodern climate of respect for the belief systems of all cultures to entertain the idea that some beliefs are demonstrably false and others, whether true or false, lead to manifestly harmful actions. We are not supposed to talk about the evolution of scientific ideas or
about progress in the Western world, since that is a colonialist way of
thinking. If it is simply "the white man's burden, medicalized"[23] to urge
African families living in the United States not to genitally mutilate their
daughters, or to attempt to educate Mien mothers about the harms of
burning their babies, then we are doomed to permit ethical relativism to
overwhelm common sense.

The Multicultural Health Care Team

Further complicating the ethics of cultural diversity is the existence of
multicultural health care teams in many, if not most, urban settings in the

United States. The following tale may be apocryphal, but I heard it in my own workplace in the Bronx, New York.

One hospital in the South Bronx has among its interns and residents many international medical graduates. They come from all parts of the world, including countries in which English is not the primary language or is not widely spoken. As a result, some of these interns and residents must communicate with their patients in a language other than their native tongue. This poses even more of a problem in a specialty like psychiatry, which relies heavily on communication for understanding a patient's condition and for a proper diagnosis and treatment. In this case the resident psychiatrist, not a native speaker of English, was examining an African-American patient. The patient told the resident: "I think I'm going bananas," and the psychiatrist wrote in the patient's chart: "Patient believes he is turning into a fruit."

Many international medical graduates obtain their medical education in countries where medical practice is still highly paternalistic. Physicians do not explain things to their patients and make little effort to communicate with them, and informed consent is all but unknown. Then they arrive in the United States and are confronted with an entirely different culture of medicine. Some find it hard to adjust, especially in cases where a patient refuses a treatment the physician believes to be indicated. In the doctor's native land, the likelihood of a patient refusing a physician's recommended treatment is rare, if it happens at all. These doctors become impatient, complain about the patients' recalcitrance and how it interferes with their work, and sometimes ridicule the way medicine in the United States grants so much power to the patient and so little to the doctor.

Does the doctrine of multiculturalism require that we be respectful of these international medical graduates' values and permit them to practice here as they were taught in their own countries? The answer is a clear "no," for two different reasons. The first is the "when in Rome" reason. Whatever the norms of practice were in their native countries, they are here now, and these are the ethical standards of medical practice in the United States. The second reason harks back to the preceding chapter, where I distinguished between norms and standards related to customary practice in the medical profession and customs that are rooted in the traditional culture of the larger society. To require international medical graduates to adhere to the ethics of medical practice in the United States does not fail to show respect for the cultural traditions of the society in which they were educated. It is, however, to reject those features of their medical training that perpetuate the sort of paternalism that is ethically unacceptable in this country today.

Suppose, however, that the behavior of international medical graduates is truly a reflection of the traditional culture from which they came. Does respect for cultural diversity then require that they be permitted the same behavior here as they would be in their native land? The answer can only be given on a case-by-case basis, but one example is telling.

The situation occurred in a large, West-coast urban hospital. The medical service included two residents from the same country but from different ethnic groups that have considerable rivalry and frequent hostility. The senior resident was a woman and the junior resident a man. In their country of origin, women are viewed as inferior to men and are always treated as subordinates. In this case, the junior resident refused to follow the instructions of the senior resident and invoked both of these reasons: "In my country, a man can refuse to take orders from a woman; it is humiliating to be told what to do by a female" and "I cannot let this ___ person tell me, a ___, what to do." The junior resident did not, in fact, respond as he should have to the senior resident's instructions, and this had repercussions on the care of patients for whom they were both responsible.

Some doctors in the hospital where this occurred thought they might have to accept these aspects of a multicultural workforce, recognizing that the cultural practices of their native country were so deep-rooted that it would be unreasonable to ask the junior resident to try to adapt to our country's dictates of antidiscrimination. Other doctors had no doubt that the behavior of the junior resident was totally unacceptable and could not be tolerated in an American hospital. The junior resident would either have to shape up or ship out.

I do not know if anyone put forth the even stronger view that the discriminatory practice in these physicians' native country is ethically wrong. To hold that members of one sex or one religion are inferior to another and to treat them as such is an ethically unacceptable form of behavior wherever it may occur. That people behave that way and the majority accepts it does not make it right. Contrary to Ruth Benedict's statement, morality is *not* just a "convenient term" for socially approved habits. At the most fundamental level, morality is a system that dictates how people ought and ought not to treat one another.

Multiculturalism, as defined at the beginning of this chapter, appears to embrace ethical relativism and yet is logically inconsistent with relativism. The second half of the definition states that multiculturalism "insists that all cultural groups be treated with respect and as equals." What does this imply with regard to cultural groups that oppress or fail to respect other cultural groups? Must the cultural groups that violate the mandate to treat all cultural groups with respect and as equals be respected themselves? It is impossible to insist that all such groups be treated with respect and as equals and at the same time accept any particular group's attitude toward and treatment of another group as inferior. Every cultural group contains subgroups within the culture: old and young, women and men, people with and people without disabilities. Are the cultural groups that discriminate against women or people with disabilities to be respected equally with those that do not?

What multiculturalism does not say is whether all of the beliefs and practices of all cultural groups must be equally respected. It is one thing to require that cultural, religious, and ethnic groups be treated as equals; that conforms to the principle of justice as equality. It is quite another thing to say that any cultural practice whatever of any group is to be tolerated and respected equally. This latter view is a statement of extreme ethical relativism. If multiculturalists endorse the principle of justice as equality, however, they must recognize that normative ethical relativism entails the illogical consequence of toleration and acceptance of numerous forms of injustice in those cultures that oppress women and religious and ethnic minorities.

Notes

1. Blaine J. Fowers and Frank C. Richardson, "Why Is Multiculturalism Good?" *American Psychologist*, Vol. 51, No. 6 (1996), p. 609.

2. Leslie J. Blackhall, Sheila T. Murphy, Gelya Frank, Vicki Michel, and Stanley Azen, "Ethnicity and Attitudes Toward Patient Autonomy," *Journal of the American Medical Association*, Vol. 274, No. 10 (1995), pp. 820–825.

3. Mirto Ojito, "Ritual Use of Mercury Prompts Testing of Children for Illness," *New York Times* (December 14, 1997), p. 49, quote from p. 55.

4. Joseph A. Carrese and Lorna A. Rhodes, "Western Bioethics on the Navajo Reservation: Benefit or Harm?" *Journal of the American Medical Association*, Vol. 274, No. 10 (1995), pp. 826–829.

5. Carrese and Rhodes, p. 828.

6. Carrese and Rhodes, p. 829.

7. Barbara Crossette, "Mutilation Seen as Risk for the Girls of Immigrants," *New York Times* (March 23, 1998), A3.

8. Celia W. Dugger, "Tug of Taboos: African Genital Rite vs. U.S. Law," *New York Times* (December 12, 1996), p. 1.

9. Dugger, pp. 1, 9.

10. Dugger, p. 9.

11. Dugger, p. 9.

12. Renée Brant, "Child Abuse or Acceptable Cultural Norms: Child Psychiatrist's Response," *Ethics & Behavior*, Vol. 5, No. 3 (1995): pp. 284–287.

13. Brant, pp. 285–286.

14. Brant, p. 287.

15. Gail Elizabeth Wyatt, "Ethical Issues in Culturally Relevant Interventions," *Ethics & Behavior*, Vol. 5, No. 3 (1995), pp. 288–290.

16. Wyatt, p. 289.

17. Tony Martin, "Cultural Contexts," *Ethics & Behavior*, Vol. 5, No. 3 (1995), pp. 290–292.

18. Martin, p. 291.

19. Martin, p. 291.

20. "Culture, Healing, and Professional Obligations," *Hastings Center Report*, Vol. 23, No. 4 (1993), p. 15.

21. Joseph Carrese, Commentary, "Culture, Healing, and Professional Obligations," p. 16.

22. Kate Brown and Andrew Jameton, Commentary, "Culture, Healing, and Professional Obligations," p. 17.

23. Soheir Morsey, "Safeguarding Women's Bodies: The White Man's Burden Medicalized," *Medical Anthropological Quarterly*, Vol. 5, No. 1 (1991), pp. 19–23.

6

Death

and

Birth

EVERY culture has customs, norms, rituals, and ethical require-ments and prohibitions surrounding death. Practices that would be considered routine or morally neutral in one society or group may be prohibited in another. Autopsy is one example. Although family members in the United States sometimes refuse to consent to a physician's request to perform an autopsy, no cultural stigma surrounds this practice. In Orthodox Jewish medical ethics, however, autopsy is strictly forbidden, and in Japan it is considered a violation of the taboo against violence to the body, which causes imbalance.[1] As the criteria for determining death have shifted over the past 30 years from cessation of heart and lung activity to the cessation of brain waves, the very concept of death has been scrutinized and debated. Nevertheless, brain death as a criterion remains unacceptable to some, both within societies and cross-culturally.

In the United States and Europe, disagreement and debate continue regarding the ethical acceptability of physician-assisted suicide and active euthanasia. Although both withholding and withdrawing life supports from patients have gained general acceptance, what is ethically right remains unsettled in a variety of specific circumstances. Removal of life supports from permanently comatose patients who never made their wishes known generates ethical arguments for and against. Some would allow for withdrawal of all life-prolonging measures, except artificial nutrition and hydration; others would allow withdrawal of all life supports but only on condition that the patient be permanently unconscious or terminally ill. Still others would allow relatives to make decisions to cease treatment of patients who are severely demented but not terminally ill.

The Roman Catholic position is frequently misunderstood as holding that it is always wrong to withhold or withdraw life supports that would result in the death of the person. The Catholic doctrine does permit rejection of life-prolonging treatments deemed "extraordinary." This derives from the statement of Pope Pius XII delivered in 1957, in which the Pope said that we are normally obliged to use only ordinary means to preserve life and that "a more strict obligation would be too burdensome for most men and would render the attainment of the higher, more important good too difficult."[2] Although this dictum makes it clear that physicians need not do everything possible to preserve and prolong life, it does not provide any criteria for distinguishing the "ordinary" from the "extaordinary." The use of these terms has fallen out of favor in the past decade or so because there is no agreement among health care professionals about which treatments should be classified under which category.

Different views on when it is permissible to end a life or to hasten death coexist in pluralistic societies like the United States and many European countries. The reason they can coexist comfortably is that public policy (so far, at least) does not require that lives be ended or death be hastened in opposition to the wishes of an individual patient or the patient's family. I say "so far" because there have been attempts by some doctors and hospitals to remove life supports from patients despite refusals by patients' families, but these attempts have not been upheld in courts. Some physicians have used their judgments of "medical futility" as grounds for removing patients from ventilators, even when a spouse or parent expressed the wish for the patient's life to be prolonged. What has prevailed so far is respect for the autonomy of the patient or the decision-making authority of the patient's family. Although this permissive stance offends people in our society who belong to "right to life" groups, it certainly does not impose on them or on anyone else an unwanted "death sentence." Ethical beliefs about when it is permissible to end life or hasten death differ substantially, and in pluralistic societies law and ethics respect these diverse views. What does this imply for the doctrine of ethical relativism?

One thing it does *not* mean is that ethical relativism follows logically from cultural diversity. Although some (but surely not all) religious faiths or denominations prohibit certain actions that would hasten or bring about death, views on ending life and hastening death in pluralist societies like the United States do not adhere strictly to ethnic or even religious lines. The doctrine of ethical relativism that relies on cultural traditions as the foundation for morality is therefore largely irrelevant to debates about when life may be ended or death hastened. The underlying and shared fundamental principle is respect for persons or, more broadly, respect for family autonomy. Adherence to the competent patient's wish to terminate treatment is accepted by all but members of religious faiths that prohibit hastening death, such as Orthodox Judaism. But there is universal opposition to terminating life-sustaining treatment of a competent patient who expresses a wish to continue the treatment. That would violate the patient's right to life in the true meaning of the phrase.

In this context, then, the conclusion seems inescapable that some things are relative, others are not. Beliefs about the circumstances in which it is permissible to terminate life-sustaining treatment are arguable, and there is no single, right position. Situations vary from patient to patient, from illness to illness. As long as individuals are not forced to accept the beliefs of others that diverge from their own, then no one's rights are violated and no one's interests are harmed. The "respect for persons" principle provides a deeper ethical justification for this variation in beliefs about ending life and hastening death.

It would be a mistake, however, to conclude that "respect for persons" is a universally accepted principle when it comes to an individual's decision about terminating life-prolonging treatment. The exception lies in religious dictates that some would place higher than the secular ethical principle that permits competent individuals to decide about life-prolonging treatments. Individuals who adhere to religious doctrines such as the Orthodox Jewish prohibition against withholding or withdrawing life supports cannot be required to adopt the secular view that grants patients the right to terminate unwanted medical treatment. "Respect for persons," in the form of religious toleration, mandates that religious opponents of individual choice in matters of life and death have their wishes respected. At the same time, they should not be permitted to impose those views on others in a society that promotes religious freedom.

Given the diverse beliefs about matters of life and death that exist within countries in which people share predominant cultural values, it is not surprising to find at least as much diversity across regions and cultures of the world. Individuals, religious faiths, and special interest groups in multicultural societies embrace positions ranging from an affirmative obligation to maintain life whenever possible to the opposite end of the spectrum where active euthanasia would be tolerated or encouraged. The justification for permitting or prohibiting the hastening of death has significant analogies across cultures or religious faiths, but the underlying universal permits patients to decide, based on their own ethical or religious beliefs. Diverse cultural beliefs about the definition of death itself are of greater interest for our purposes because they have consequences for public policy regarding organ transplantation.

Definition of Death and Organ Transplantation

The criterion of "brain death" was introduced as an alternative to the cessation of heart and lung functions to facilitate the harvesting of organs for transplantation. Solid organs deteriorate rapidly after blood ceases to circulate, but placing a patient on a ventilator can enable the blood to continue to circulate even after brain activity has stopped. The determination that brain death is the death of the person allows the organs to be removed from patients who have died, despite their artificially maintained beating heart and breathing lungs.

Based on the interpretation of ancient holy texts from which contemporary Orthodox Jewish views are derived, the predominant Orthodox Jewish position rejects the brain death criterion. A Native-American perspective understands death to be a complete stoppage of the vital functions of the body and therefore also rejects cessation of brain wave activity as the criterion of the death of the person. A fierce debate has raged in Japan over the ethical acceptability of brain death, a battle that one writer describes as "a kind of Japanese counterpart of the abortion issue in the United States in terms of its rancor."[3]

A widely accepted assumption is that the grounds for denying brain death and organ transplantation in Japan stem from the traditional Japanese view of life and death.[4] That traditional view holds that human beings are completely integrated mind–body units. Because the unit persists after death, removing an organ from a dead body is viewed as disturbing the spiritual and corporal unity and not simply altering the physical body. The same traditional view underlies the abhorrence of autopsies in Japan. Japanese tradition has roots in Buddhist, Shinto, and Confucian sources. Buddhist and Shinto thought maintains that the mind–body unity of human beings extends to all living things. Death disturbs the rhythm of all living things and therefore should not be hastened. Unlike the United States, where people have come to reject the use of technology to prolong the dying process, Japanese people are more concerned that life not end prematurely and so they seek to maintain dying rituals.[5]

What is more, the Confucian tradition stresses the idea of filial piety and family relationships. Because the body is derived from one's parents, this results in a prohibition against harming one's body. Buddhism also holds that consciousness is not located solely in the brain, so the death of the brain does not extinguish consciousness and therefore cannot be regarded as the death of the person. Still another Buddhist belief rounds out the traditional opposition to organ transplantation. Because the extension of an individual's life by means of receiving an organ transplant depends on the death of the other person, this mode of life extension is regarded as unnatural and unethical.[6] Many rituals surround death in Japan, and the society attaches great importance to these rituals. The use of the brain death criterion and the subsequent harvesting of organs intrude on these traditional rituals and are seen as violations of important cultural components of death and dying.[7]

These traditional beliefs only partially explain the opposition to the brain death criterion and to organ transplantation in Japan today. One writer says that the number of people who adhere to the traditional view of death is now a minority in Japan.[8] Japanese people who have had organ transplants from brain-dead donors in other countries have been warmly welcomed in the mass media in Japan. However, it remains the case that transplantation of vital organs from dead bodies in Japan is rare.[9] Outwardly, at least, organ transplantation from brain-dead donors is still banned. The explanation that does not rely on traditional beliefs points to the fear that organs will be removed prematurely and that transplants will be performed under unethical circumstances. Further evidence that it is this fear, rather than the traditional religious thinking, that has caused the continued ban on removing organs from brain-dead donors is the fact that corneas and kidneys are transplanted from brain-dead bodies. Removal of the heart from a still-living donor would obviously cause the death of the patient, but removal of kidneys or corneas would not. Fear of premature organ removal is certainly not unique to the Japanese context, as it has been a prominent concern in many places where organ transplantation is performed.

A different, culturally relative explanation has been offered for the reluctance to accept brain death in Japan. A cultural feature of contemporary Japanese society is said to be "mutual dependency and ostracism."[10] In contrast to the Western, pluralist approach to bioethics, this feature of Japanese culture seeks to attain consensus. Once brain death had met with critical reception in Japan, it became something to be ostracized. In the Japanese society of "mutual dependency," pluralism is not allowed. This is Japanese "morality," which would not permit a viewpoint from Western bioethics to be accepted in its original form. Although no one suggests that Western society was somehow seeking to impose its contemporary view of brain death on Japanese society, some in Japan continue to voice the view that "all evils come from the West."[11] A minority opinion expressed in a Parliamentary study of brain death sought to uphold the traditional Japanese perspective, and that minority opposed the acceptance of brain death. The group that rejects Western ideas sees Japanese tradition and culture as superior to Western materialism and is likely to reject anything that is Western in origin for that reason.

But in the Parliamentary study, the majority did support a Western position on brain death: People who adhere to the traditional view of death should have their wishes respected, and organs should be taken from brain-dead individuals only when those individuals have accepted brain death and indicated their desire to donate their organs. This solution, if adopted as law in Japan, will no doubt lead to the same shortage of organs for donation that persists in the United States. Only a minority of people who are suitable donors have indicated their willingness to be a donor, and even then, if the family objects, transplant surgeons will not harvest the organs. A 1992 commission report in Japan permits the individual and family to make a choice between the cession of the function of the entire brain and the heart–lung criterion as the basis for determining the death of the individual.[12]

One inescapable conclusion is that traditional Japanese beliefs have given way to beliefs influenced by Western practices; but advancing medical technology is also a contributing cause of change. Many of the advanced medical technologies, such as reproductive technology, have altered the traditional Japanese view of life and death. By way of contrast, it

is instructive to see what has happened with the passage of the organ donation act in the Philippines.

A controversy erupted in the Philippines when the press reported a
case in which doctors declared a patient brain dead and removed organs
for transplantation from his body without first having succeeded in locating the patient's relatives. The doctors' behavior was in accordance with
provisions of the Act Authorizing the Legacy or Donation of All or Part of a
Human Body After Death for Specified Purposes. The Act includes two alternative definitions of death: absence of unaided cardiac and respiratory
functions and irreversible cessation of all brain functions.[13]

The determination of the death of the patient whose organs were removed in the controversial case was based on the brain-death criterion of
the law. However, Philippine society has not fully accepted this concept of
death because of deep-seated values, practices, and rituals associated with
death and dying. Other features of the Act include a 48-hour waiting period to exert reasonable efforts to locate the nearest relative, following
which the head of a hospital or other designated official may authorize the
removal of organs for transplantation.

A rather subtle consideration of traditional morality enters into the
picture of organ donation in the Philippines. The dead person whose organs are removed is not in a position to make a proper "donation" in an act
that stems from the right sort of moral motivation. The relevant concept in
the traditional Filipino value system is known as *kusang loob*. For an act to
have moral worth it must be done out of *kusang loob*, an idea similar to
free will but not exactly the same. If a person needs to be told what to do,
or is coerced into performing an action, the act does not come out of *kusang loob*. To have moral worth, an action must also be done without an-
ticipation of reward or personal gain and not purely out of a sense of duty.

The implications for the morality of organ donation are rather
straightforward. If a person is not in a position to act from the proper moral
motivation, that is, out of *kusang loob*, it is better for that action not to have
been done at all. Presumably, then, only if a person had signed an organ
donation card, done so in an uncoerced manner and not purely out of a
sense of duty, would the donation qualify as being done out of *kusang loob*.
Perhaps also the prospective donor would have to designate a particular

recipient or group of potential recipients, because *kusang loob* requires people to have genuine feelings for the beneficiaries of their actions. Because these conditions are rarely fulfilled in the Philippines (or elsewhere, for that matter), organ donation remains a problematic ethical concern for those whose moral beliefs rely on the concept of *kusang loob*.

What follows from this picture for ethical relativism? Should we conclude that the medical practice of organ transplantation is ethically wrong in the Philippines because of the value attached to the concept of *kusang loob* but ethically right elsewhere as long as the proper safeguards are followed? That would be a misunderstanding of the Filipino doctrine. It is not the practice of organ transplantation that the doctrine rejects but, rather, instances in which the donation of organs lacks the proper motivation.

However, the traditional moral concept of *kusang loob* is not the only relevant ethical concern. Filipinos are worried about the possibility of exploitation stemming from a bias against economically disadvantaged members of the society. People in the lower social classes are more likely to end up as accident victims who remain unidentified for some time. Poorer people have less access to newspapers, radio, or television, which serve as aids in identifying accident victims. In contrast, those who benefit from organ transplantation are the wealthier classes. They are the only ones who can afford the cost of transplant surgery in the Philippines.

With the advent of organ transplantation in the Philippines, the Organ Donation Act was crafted in a manner designed to shield doctors from civil liability or criminal prosecution. It was also designed to enlarge the pool of potential recipients of organs by including the 48-hour provision after which the removal of organs could be authorized without permission of a family member. A philosopher who wrote about this general situation in the Philippines concluded that "the transfer of medical technology should be accompanied by appropriate mechanisms for dealing with the accompanying transfer of values."[14] In particular, people should have an opportunity to receive new technology with *kusang loob*.

This conclusion does not state that organ transplantation itself is wrong in the Philippines. Rather, it seems that the way the practice has been legally authorized and medically implemented creates problems.

Perhaps the features of the Organ Donation Act are biased too much in the direction of physicians' ability to procure organs and are insufficient to adequately protect the donors. People in the Philippines may be worried (whether justifiably or not), as apparently many Japanese people are, about coercion in the form of social pressure, exploitation, and premature removal of organs from the not yet dead. These fears have little to do with cultural differences and much to do with the universal dread of being declared dead when one is still alive or having one's death hastened to harvest organs to save the life of another.

Nevertheless, the Filipino concept of *kusang loob* is a feature of a moral system in that culture that does not appear to have an exact counterpart in our own society, at least not with respect to organ donation. *Kusang loob* falls under the category of moral motivation, an aspect of ethical behavior that may legitimately differ from one society to another and is therefore an example of one of the things that turns out to be relative. The application of this concept to organ donation yields the result that organ donation itself is neither morally right nor morally wrong, but its rightness or wrongness depends (among other things) on the moral motivation of the individual whose organs are harvested for transplantation. This marks a cultural and ethical difference from organ donation in other cultures where a donation need not stem from a particular moral motivation. This difference is not at the level of fundamental ethical principles, so it does not confirm the proposition that ethical principles vary from one culture to the next with no deeper underlying principles. Rather, it confirms the much more limited thesis that some things are relative from one culture to the next. According to the traditional Filipino culture, the motive from which an action is performed must be of a certain type, as shown by the example of organ donations.

Feticide and Infanticide

Almost as many rituals, customs, prescriptions, and prohibitions exist regarding birth as surround death. For the same reason I have chosen not to explore cultural variations in beliefs and prohibitions regarding euthanasia and suicide, I choose not to rehearse all viewpoints in the classic debate about the ethics of abortion. When there is as much variation within a country or culture (Western culture, in this case) as there is cross-culturally, it is beside the point to examine ethical relativism as a derivative of cultural diversity. The "classic" debate about the ethics of abortion arises out of different views about when life acquires a moral status. Whether described in terms of the "personhood" of the fetus, the time at which the gestating embryo or fetus acquires moral standing, or the "right to life" of a fertilized ovum or viable fetus, the classic debate stems from a range of different positions on the moral status of intrauterine life.

It is of some interest, however, to look at a position on the ethics of abortion that emanates from a completely different world view. The world view of the Nso' people of the Bamenda Highlands of Kamerun is described by an African scholar as guided by the taboo against harvesting premature crops or fruits.[15] Among the Nso' people it is taboo to harvest any crop before it has been certified mature enough for harvesting and appropriate ritual ceremonies performed. This taboo stems from a belief about the consequences of picking immature crops: Such actions are believed to bring personal misfortune. The same taboo is the basis for prohibiting sex with girls before adolescence and for a prohibition against killing pregnant animals. It extends, as well, to abortion of a human fetus.

From our Western perspective, it would appear that picking an unripe melon or killing a pregnant goat in the Nso' culture is as serious an offense as sex with minors because all three actions stem from the same taboo and the same belief about the consequences of such actions. But it may be a mistake to judge the seriousness of such transgressions from our Western perspective. A "therapeutic" abortion could be justified by the Nso' beliefs if, for example, the life of the pregnant woman was at risk because of the pregnancy. This is because of the underlying belief that an evil spirit may have disguised itself and lodged in the woman's womb under the pretext of being an unborn child. The appropriate ritual would then be to dislodge the intruding evil sprit by means of rites and medicaments. What is critical here are the beliefs that underlie the justification for abortion. An unborn baby is like an unripe melon, and so the taboo extends to plucking either before maturity. If, instead of an unborn baby an evil spirit resides within the woman's womb, the prohibition against harvesting premature crops obviously does not apply.

An additional aspect of the Nso' attitude toward killing fetuses and infants is that, whereas nontherapeutic abortion is considered wrong, infanticide is permissible in the case of a pregnancy resulting from incest. The Nso' believe that incest pollutes the entire family and lineage, and if it occurs an elaborate purification rite is required. (The incest taboo in this culture extends far beyond first-degree relatives, unlike many societies, and includes prohibition against sex between cousins up to the fifth degree.) If a child is conceived as a result of an incestuous union, the infant is immediately killed after birth. The man and woman who committed the act are, however, considered free of the stigma once the purification rite is carried out. Incest is not a capital offense in this culture, but adultery is. However, if a pregnancy results from an adulterous union the woman's life is spared until the baby is born, after which the mother is clubbed to death. When a leader was asked, "Why not kill her sooner?" he replied, "What Nso' man would pluck an unripe melon!?"[16]

There is no way to make a cross-cultural ethical judgment of the Nso' ethical practices regarding feticide and infanticide without questioning the system of beliefs on which those practices rest. That system includes beliefs about presumed "matters of fact" (the personal misfortune believed to be a consequence of harvesting premature crops or fruits) as well as comparative ethical judgments: a woman who commits adultery must be punished by death, while the life of her unborn baby must be preserved; an infant resulting from an incestuous union must be killed, but it is wrong to kill a fetus unless the life of the mother is in jeopardy. These assessments of the comparative worth of the life of an infant versus a fetus, or that of a woman who transgresses the moral law versus that of her unborn baby, diverge from our Western scale of values. Is it legitimate to judge our scale of comparative worth to be morally right and the Nso' values to be morally wrong?

We have first to recognize that these cross-cultural differences are no greater, in certain respects, than ethical values that exist side by side within the Western culture that Americans on both continents and Europeans have in common. Our culture is sometimes characterized as

"Judeo-Christian" in its moral origins, but some of the differences within the dominant Western culture are as great as the differences between us and the Nso' people. An illustration from secular rather than religious-based views is the divergence in ethical beliefs about capital punishment.

The United States is the only Western industrialized country that practices capital punishment. Europeans generally consider state-authorized taking of human life to be barbaric or, at least, a product of backward, unenlightened thinking. Canada, Australia, Hungary, and the Czech Republic are among other countries that have abolished capital punishment. How, opponents ask, can a civilized nation prohibit torture of criminals on the grounds that it violates human rights and yet sanction the killing of people who have committed similar crimes?

The Nso' people treat adultery as a crime punishable by death, and we in the United States do not. Islamic law also contains the death penalty for adultery, and it is imposed in some fundamentalist Islamic societies. The difference between those in the United States who believe in capital punishment and the beliefs in the Nso' culture and Islamic societies is much narrower than the difference between supporters and opponents of capital punishment in the United States. The former is a dispute about which actions should be punishable by death, whereas the latter is a more profound disagreement about whether death should ever serve as punishment for transgression against secular or religious law.

Or consider the exceptions that most organized groups opposed to abortion rights would allow. Virtually every group opposed to abortion makes an exception in cases where the life of the woman is at stake. That pits fetal life against the life of an adult person and concludes that in a case of conflict the woman's life is worth more. But how can opponents of abortion justify exceptions in cases of rape and incest? If a fertilized ovum has the same right to life as a person born alive, the way in which the embryo came into existence should make no difference. Opponents of abortion who allow for these exceptions would not sanction the killing of an infant or a 5-year-old child who was the product of rape or incest. How, then, can they condone abortion in cases in which the existence of embryos and fetuses is a consequence of the same acts? The Nso' practice of killing an infant whose conception results from incest is on a par with permitting abor-

tion in cases of rape and incest. In both cultures, killing in such cases is
sanctioned as a function of how the life came into existence. Again, the
difference in ethical beliefs between opponents and proponents of a
woman's right to abortion within our Western culture are greater than the
difference between opponents of abortion here, who would permit killing
a fetus conceived through incest, and the Nso' people who kill a newborn
infant resulting from incest.

Sex Determination

The thought of women having abortions to choose the sex of their future
children fills many people with revulsion. But for individuals or entire societies for whom killing a fetus bears little, if any, moral relation to killing
an infant or child, other factors determine whether it is ethical to select the
sex of one's child.[17] The introduction of amniocentesis, ultrasound, and
other methods of detecting the sex of the fetus prior to birth has led to a
burgeoning industry in India of sex determination followed by abortion of
female fetuses. But before prenatal diagnosis was available, and in parts of
India today where women either do not have access to or cannot afford
medical tests, female infanticide has been another manifestation of the
strong preference for sons.

The social and cultural bases for son preference in India, China, and
other parts of Asia are long-standing and deeply entrenched. Religious traditions and economic circumstances drive the preference for sons beyond
that in most other countries. In both India and China the family name is
passed down through sons, who are also financially responsible for supporting their parents in old age. In India, a precept of the Hindu religion
holds that a sonless father cannot achieve salvation, and a significant
Hindu funeral rite can only be performed by male children for their fathers. An analogous tradition in China stems from ancient Confucian precepts that require a son to perform ancestral worship ceremonies.

The most striking determinant of son preference in India in recent
times is probably the dowry system, which has escalated from providing a
few necessities of domestic life for the newly married couple to a demand

on the bride's family for vast sums of money and increasing numbers of consumer goods such as color TVs and VCRs. These demands continue even after the marriage, and the consequences of a failure to meet the demands can include ejection of the woman from the marriage and even her murder by her husband's family.[18]

Economic factors evidently provide a major incentive today for a decision to abort female fetuses; nevertheless, the underlying cultural tradition of son preference remains a strong determinant. In one case, a middle-class Indian woman who was pregnant with her third child underwent prenatal diagnosis for the purpose of sex selection. She already had two daughters and planned to abort if the fetus was another female. The woman's husband ran a family business, and they were reasonably well off. The woman said that it was not that she and her husband could not afford another girl, nor was it that they did not love their daughters. Instead, social attitudes were so strong that she was made to feel inadequate having only daughters.

The woman told an interviewer: "Our society makes you feel so bad if you don't have a son. . . . Especially when I go out for parties, people say, 'How many children?' and I say, 'Two girls,' and they say, 'Oh, too bad, no boy.' And I feel very bad." This woman and her husband were both Roman Catholics, relatively rare in India. She said, "Being a Catholic, it's the only sin I commit." But, she added: "When this test is here and everybody is doing it, why shouldn't we have what we want?"[19]

In China, ancient Confucian ideology continues to influence the strong preference for sons, especially the first-born child. In addition to the need for sons to maintain the family line and to perform crucial ancestral rituals, males are held to be smarter and stronger than females. Despite a law in modern China dictating that parental support is the duty of all children, males are still held responsible for the support of parents in old age. In contrast, women are not available for the care of their own elderly parents because once they are married their productive and reproductive labors benefit their husband's families.[20]

A report published in June 1986 in *India Today* estimated that 6,000 female babies had been poisoned to death during the preceding decade in the district surrounding the town of Madurai in Tamil Nadu.[21] Methods of infanticide included feeding the baby the sticky white milk of a poisonous plant or cow's milk mixed with sleeping pills. One mother of a day-old baby who had been killed by giving her the milk from the plant was reported as saying, "We felt very bad. . . . But at the same time, suppose she had lived? It was better to save her from a lifetime of suffering."[22] The mother of another couple who had had their second daughter killed said, "Abortion is costly . . . and you have to rest at home. So instead of spending money and losing income, we prefer to deliver the child and kill it."[23]

At least for some people in countries where a strong son preference exists, infanticide is a reasonable (if not preferred) alternative to aborting female fetuses. Even for the most strenuous opponents of abortion, killing an infant is still a morally worse act than killing a fetus. But some radical feminists apparently believe that female feticide is morally equivalent to infanticide. One Indian feminist wrote a response to an article of mine published in an Indian journal of medical ethics. In my article I said that from any ethical perspective other than an extreme right to life position, aborting previable fetuses is ethically preferable to killing full-term infants after birth.[24] The respondent wrote that my formulation "blurs gender perspective" and added, "We will not say that female foeticide is ethically preferable to female infanticide. Both victimize the woman. Our response is: Eliminate inequality, not women."[25]

The difference between my conclusion about the wrong involved in female feticide, as compared with infanticide, and the very different view expressed by the Indian feminist had nothing to do with the cultural relativity of values in our respective cultures. The difference lay in her adoption of the radical feminist agenda that begins and ends with one interpretation of what gender justice requires and my multiply principled approach to ethics, which incorporates a broader notion of gender justice and at the same time distinguishes between the moral status of a fetus and that of an infant.

Both India and China have enacted legal prohibitions of practices contributing to abortion for the purpose of choosing male children over females. As of 1995, selective elimination of a fetus because of its sex is an offense under the Indian Penal Code, the Medical Termination of Pregnancy Act, the Constitution of India, and a number of state laws. In spite of all these laws, however, the practice has continued to thrive.[26] The enactment of prohibitionist legislation was largely a result of the work of a nongovernmental organization, the Forum Against Sex-Determination and Sex-Preselection (FASDSP), that campaigned vigorously against sex determination. But the law has not changed the attitudes of the Indian population regarding their preference for sons. What prohibition has done is driven the practice of sex determination underground. Prenatal diagnosis is done in a private office or clinic, and the patient is discharged in a few hours. Doctors communicate the results orally and the patient then decides whether to go for an abortion.

Evidence is lacking whether legal prohibition of prenatal diagnosis for the purpose of sex selection has led to a higher incidence of female infanticide in India. One thing is clear, however: Those who are financially better off can readily avail themselves of the diagnostic test but poor women cannot. The tests used to be carried out in public hospitals as well as in private clinics. Because poor women cannot afford private practitioners they use the public health care institutions. But after the laws were passed, physicians in the public hospitals ceased to perform prenatal diagnosis for the purpose of sex determination, with the result that poor women were left with three undesirable alternatives. They could further impoverish themselves by selling possessions or forgo food and other necessities for themselves or their daughters; they could continue the pregnancy and if the baby turns out female, perform infanticide (despite its illegality); or they could keep having children until they had a son or the desired number of sons.

Ample evidence is available to document the death of female children from starvation and neglect. A Unicef report from 1996 notes that malnutrition is one of the major causes of death of female children. In south Asia, for example, it is common for men to eat the most and the best, leaving the women and children to eat the last and the least. The mother then feeds her sons most of what is left, at the expense of her own and her daughters' nutritional well-being.

In China, Fujian province banned prenatal diagnosis for the purpose of sex determination in 1996. Demographic data showed a ratio of 100 females to 115.4 males in this province, and the law was passed to try to counteract the growing imbalance in the sex ratio. Penalties would be leveled both at the physician who conducted prenatal tests for this purpose and the women who have aborted a fetus after prenatal sex determination. Physicians risk losing their medical license, and women would be denied official permission to give birth for 5 years.[27] Based on the difficulty China has had enforcing its one-child policy, it is doubtful whether it will prove possible to detect violations and enforce this new law.

This digression has led us away from the focus on ethical relativism. To bring us back, we may frame the issue in the following terms. Can actions intended to determine the sex of one's child, based on a strong preference for sons, be condemned in some societies but considered ethically acceptable in others? It is clear that when the means of determining the sex of the child involves abortion or infanticide, the major ethical concern becomes the method used to attain the desired end. A costly and highly technical technique already exists that would not involve abortion. That method is sex-selective embryo transfer, rarely used even in technologically advanced societies and certainly not an option in India. The future will no doubt see the perfection of sex-selective insemination, a technique that will bypass all concerns related to abortion and the destruction of embryos. For now, we can contemplate abortion of female fetuses as the only practical method of sex determination. But the question on which to focus is whether preventing the birth of female children is an ethically acceptable practice. Once it becomes possible to separate sperm to ensure that a child of the desired sex is conceived, the ethical issue will no longer involve abortion but will focus entirely on the ethics of sex selection.

Although sex determination is currently prohibited by the Medical Termination of Pregnancy Act in India, we may still consider the ethics of the practice, just as people debated the ethics of abortion in the United States before and after *Roe v. Wade*. The presence of a law may be related to the ethics of an action or practice but does not alone determine its rightness or wrongness from a moral point of view.

Is it the preference itself for males over females, sons rather than daughters, that critics of sex determination find morally objectionable? Is it solely the means used to attain the desired end—abortion or infanticide—that is the source of ethical concern? Or is it the consequences for a region, a country, or even the world of an imbalance in the sex ratio that is worrisome? The answer appears to be "all of the above," depending on the form of ethical argument and the underlying assumptions made by critics of sex determination.

The Indian FASDSP set out the following six reasons for opposing sex determination: (1) it devalues the female sex; (2) it reinforces current attitudes and practices that discriminate against girl children and women; (3) it objectifies women by treating them only as son-producing machines, raw material for invasive technologies and scientific experimentation; (4) it encourages husband and relatives to place tremendous psychological pressure on women to prove their social worth by producing sons; (5) it converts healthy women into patients at the mercy of the commercial interest in the medical market; and (6) it produces an imbalance in the sex ratio.[28]

None of these reasons for the condemnation of sex determination appeals to traditional values or cultural practices in India in support of the ethical conclusion. Ironically, the opposite is true. Opponents of sex determination within India are seeking to reject the long-standing traditional preference for sons. They are also eager to reject the social system according to which sons are responsible for the support of their elderly parents and the tradition of dowry that is placing increasing economic hardships on middle-class as well as poor families when they seek to marry off their daughters. In this situation, the strongest opponents of traditional values and customs come from within the society and have succeeded in achieving a legal prohibition.

Where, then, is the ethical relativism in this picture? The people in India who are most opposed to sex determination not only reject their own culture's value of son preference, but argue for a universal ethics based on gender equality. A majority of the reasons cited by the FASDSP group appeal to concepts of justice held to be universally valid, such as the wrongs involved in sex discrimination, objectification and commodification of women, and devaluing and oppressing members of the female sex. These are values that are not peculiarly Eastern or Western and are certainly not rooted in the traditional culture of India, especially the Hindu caste system. Western ethical principles can and do support the idea of gender equality and oppose devaluation and oppression of individuals or classes of persons.

Just as ethical principles can be used in support of the FASDSP agenda in India, so too can they be used to criticize that agenda. Following my visit to India,[29] I came to believe that the problem of sex determination in that country has all the marks of a genuine ethical dilemma. As is true of many ethical dilemmas, this one arises out of a conflict between ethical principles. During my brief visit I interviewed physicians, researchers, activists, social scientists, and public health leaders. These included numerous people who defended the legislation prohibiting sex determination as well as some who questioned its efficacy and cited its negative consequences for Indian women from the poorer classes. I also consulted articles and books, some provided to me by people I spoke with in India and others located through a literature search. The conclusion I came to did not change my judgment that sex selection is certainly an undesirable action in India and wherever else it may be practiced; nevertheless, to prohibit it by law is probably causing more harm than good to the very people it seeks to protect—members of the female sex. Here are some of the facts.

One Bombay physician who formerly performed prenatal diagnosis followed by abortion of female fetuses told me that enacting the law in his state, Maharashtra, played into the hands of unethical people. Physicians who perform amniocentesis sometimes do it unscrupulously, telling women that the fetus is a girl when it is not. Financial motivation on the part of greedy physicians, conjoined with legal prohibition, has led to a worse situation than before the ban. One physician, asked by a patient for a cheaper rate than the going rate of 5,000 rupees [about $160] for performing the prenatal test, replied: "You must go in for a reliable test. I aborted several male foetuses because the parents went to an unreliable doctor."[30] Honest and scrupulous physicians, however, will comply with the law. The Bombay doctor who had practiced sex selection before the law was enacted stated his belief that "you can't violate the law of the land," so he has ceased. He said that it was wrong to enact the law, but now it is the law and it must be respected.

Soon after the national prohibition was enacted, a professor at the

University of Delhi expressed her view that "All you are doing with this new law is giving the police a new potential for extorting bribes. Now, instead of extorting from street hawkers, they'll be extorting from doctors."[31] Before the ban, the same scholar had observed: "Female feticide is a symptom of devaluation of female lives. Unless we are able to deal with all those social and economic factors that are going into the culture of son-preference and daughter-aversion, we cannot effectively combat the killing of unwanted female fetuses."[32] This assessment agrees with the premises of the FASDSP position but comes to the opposite conclusion regarding the desirability of a law prohibiting sex determination.

I interviewed Indian women who strongly supported legislation prohibiting sex selection and others who questioned the wisdom of enacting the prohibition. Rami Chabra, the author of a book entitled *Abortion in India: An Overview*, said her background has been that of working on women's issues "forever." When our discussion turned to sex determination, she provided a brief historical overview. Back in 1977–78, when prenatal diagnosis was first introduced in India, it was discovered that women were coming in for genetic tests, obtaining information about the sex of the child, and were aborting the girl fetuses. A law was then passed banning the test for purposes of sex determination alone. She said that a question to be concerned about today is whether the rhetoric regarding "feminine feticide" will lead to questioning feticide in general, possibly then opening the door to prohibiting abortion for any reason. Abortion in India has not been accompanied by the political, ethical, and religious controversies that have occurred elsewhere, but, Rami Chabra said, a dangerous trend could begin once some legal restrictions on women's right to abortion are in place.

I asked whether the feminist groups in India recognize these dangers, and Rami said most do see the force of these arguments. She added that *feticide* is a powerful term, one that produces an emotional response. Her own fear is that other bans on abortion could emerge as a result of using this emotional terminology to argue against sex determination. Echoing the accounts of others, she said that the law has not eradicated prenatal diagnosis and abortion for the purpose of sex selection. Women are demanding it and seeking it. Rami Chabra said that women in India are not empowered enough to go along with feminist concerns without distorting their own lives. The birth of a girl child will bring about drama in the home. Do we have a right to stop such women from exercising their choices, she asked? In the face of these developments, and with more vulnerable women being denied the choice of sex determination, what is the right thing to do, she wondered: "Draw the blinders down? Or make it more available?"

In the end, Rami Chabra admitted to being torn about these issues because of the conflict of values they involve. She described her own bottom line as follows: Whenever a choice is to be made, opt for the adult woman and for her rights. In the lives of most Indian women, the attainment of feminist ideals is not possible. Therefore, the best course of action overall is to increase the woman's choice and her options in her own life. Still there is a problem: How to argue for this position and yet not reinforce the practice of sex determination? Women are so hamstrung by their personal circumstances, it is important to spend time figuring out the balances. Female infanticide, as well as neglect of girl children, has continued to increase. Thus the consequences for girl children who are born and survive are grim.

Rami Chabra's position can readily be classified as that of the liberal feminist, in contrast to the larger and much more vocal group of radical feminists who comprise the movement in India. Yet I did encounter another spokesperson for the liberal position, Nina Puri of the Family Planning Association of India. She began her thoughts on the current state of sex determination in India by noting its interrelation "with the dowry business." A woman she met at a party told her that her maid has four or five daughters. The maid has now had four or five abortions after sex determination because the fetuses were all found to be female. The maid herself described this as a "wonderful thing that is coming"—to get the son she wants. She otherwise would not be accepted by her husband or his family. Sex determination is a boon to her. In her economic bracket, the financial cost of the test and the subsequent abortion is much lower than what she would have to pay for raising a girl child. In Haryana state, where the woman lives, girls have very little premium placed on them. It is more important for people living there to be able to afford another cow. However, "a boy is a boy," Nina Puri said.

She reiterated the negative consequences for girl children that I had heard before. Girls are removed from school to give the opportunity to sons; because boys need nutrition to work in the fields, girls are given less nutrition if the family is poor. At every level, there is discrimination against girls. The biggest one is health. To pay medical bills for the health of a boy, people will sell their houses. Yet parents may not even take their daughters to the doctor when they are sick.

I asked how such social attitudes can possibly be changed. Her optimistic reply was that it may take time, but things can change. In fact, things are already changing even in the rural areas. Some couples have said, after having a girl child, that they want a sterilization. It may be rare, but at least some people are voicing this view. In such instances, Nina Puri said, she counsels them not to have the sterilization just yet. Although son preference is an attitude independent of one's status as rich or poor, educated or uneducated, changes will occur when opportunities increase for women in the work force. Many families are now very happy with two girls. If girls are eventually able to provide for their older parents, they may be valued more. Now, as they have begun to enter the work force, they are able to do so.

Along with describing the roots of these attitudes in traditional Indian culture, Nina Puri's account confirmed that culture is constantly undergoing change. She referred to what I had heard before: At last rites, the son releases the evil spirits of the parents, performing the religious duty of freeing the soul from the body. If there are no sons in the family, then a cousin-brother will do it. Traditionally, girls could not be allowed do perform this rite. But this, too, is changing: There are some women wanting to perform the last rites of their parents.

These two feminists had reached the same conclusion about sex determination based on the apparent consequences: There are benefits to individual women from the opportunity to choose the sex of their child and have the much-desired son. It provides an option they would not otherwise have. Some women who engage in the practice seem to believe that what they are doing is somehow wrong, but it is still better than the alternatives facing them. Moreover, the consequences of prohibiting the practice appear to be worse for Indian women and their girl children than what has been gained by the ban.

After interviewing liberal feminists like Nina Puri and Rami Chabra, as well as the more numerous radical feminists to whom I was introduced during my visit, I wrote down my thoughts in the article referred to earlier that was published in an Indian journal of medical ethics. My conclusion in that article was that sex determination is an ethically questionable practice for all the reasons stated by its opponents. Moreover, the long-term consequences of a severely imbalanced ratio of males to females in some societies could include an increase in male dominance and a worsening of the tendency to treat women as commodities. Nevertheless, legal prohibition restricts reproductive rights, a restriction that is undesirable everywhere and especially in countries like India and China, both of which have experienced such serious violations of the rights of women as forced sterilizations and administration of state-imposed, long-term contraception.

It would require further study and gathering of substantial amounts of evidence to draw the stronger conclusion that legal prohibition of sex determination produces more harms than benefits to women and girl children in societies with strong son preference. A growing body of evidence has begun to suggest that the harm to the society as a whole from an imbalance in the sex ratio may be the ultimate factor that determines the wrongness of sex selection.

This way of analyzing and assessing ethics and public policy relies on the actual and predicted consequences for the individuals and classes of people who stand to be affected most. Some might object to this utilitarian mode of ethical analysis, but public policy must be based on the observed and projected benefits and harms produced by a policy. Public policy that rests on ethical foundations must also take account of the rights of individuals. One of the most cherished rights in Western culture is the right of liberty, of freedom to choose, of self-determination. It is precisely this right, however, over which one prominent branch of the international feminist movement rides roughshod. In striving to implement their version of "gender justice," members of this international feminist movement discount the rights of individual women. The passage of laws in India prohibiting sex determination is only one manifestation of the view held by leading radical feminists that they know what is best for all women.

Notes

1. Emiko Ohnuki-Tierney, "Brain Death and Organ Transplantation," *Current Anthropology*, Vol. 35, No. 3 (1994), pp. 233–242.

2. Pope Pius XII, *Acta Apostolocae Sedis* 49 (1057), pp. 1031–1032.

3. Kenzo Hamano, "Human Rights and Japanese Bioethics," *Bioethics*, Vol. 11 (1997), p. 333.

4. Noritoshi Tanida, "Bioethics Is Subordinate to Morality in Japan," *Bioethics*, Vol. 10 (1996).

5. Rihito Kimura, "Japan's Dilemma with the Definition of Death," *Kennedy Institute of Ethics Journal*, Vol. 1, No. 2 (1991), 123–131.

6. Rihito Kimura, "Medical Ethics, History of: South and East Asia, Contemporary Japan," (ed.) Warren T. Reich, *Encyclopedia of Bioethics*, 2nd edition (New York: MacMillan, 1995), pp. 1496–1505.

7. Kimura, "Japan's Dilemma with the Definition of Death," pp. 123–131.

8. Tanida, p. 209.

9. Kimura, "Medical Ethics, History of: South and East Asia, Contemporary Japan," p. 1500.

10. Tanida, p. 203.

11. Tanida, p. 209.

12. Kimura, "Medical Ethics, History of: South and East Asia, Contemporary Japan," p. 1501.

13. Leonardo D. De Castro, "Transporting Values by Technology Transfer," *Bioethics*, Vol. 11, No. 3/4 (1997). The account that follows is taken from this article.

14. De Castro, p. 205.

15. Godfrey Tangwa, "Bioethics: An African Perspective," *Bioethics*, Vol. 10, No. 3 (1996), pp. 183–200.

16. Tangwa, p. 197.

17. Most of the information discussed in this section was gathered during my visit to India in March 1994 as part of my Ford Foundation project. The visit focused primarily on the issue of sex determination.

18. Elisabeth Bumiller, *May You Be theMother of a Hundred Sons: A Journey Among the Women of India* (New York: Random House, 1990), pp. 44–74.

19. Bumiller, pp. 115–116.

20. Elizabeth Moen, "Sex Selective Eugenic Abortion: Prospects in China

and India," *Issues in Reproductive and Genetic Engineering,* Vol. 4 (1991), 231–249.

21. Bumiller, p. 105.

22. Bumiller, p. 108.

23. Bumiller, pp. 108–110.

24. Ruth Macklin, "The Ethics of Sex Selection," *Medical Ethics,* Vol. 3, No. 4 (1995), pp. 61–64.

25. Vibhuti Patel, "The Ethics of Gender Justice," *Medical Ethics,* Vol. 3, No. 4 (1995), p. 66.

26. K. Kusum, "Sex Selection" (eds.) Claude Sureau and Francoise Shenfield, *Ethical Aspects of Human Reproduction* (Paris: John Libbey Eurotext, 1995), pp. 302–304.

27. "Chinese Province Bans Tests for Sex of Fetus" (Reuters), *New York Times,* June 7, 1996, A11.

28. Patel, pp. 65–66.

29. This visit was part of my Ford Foundation project on ethics and reproductive health.

30. "Female foetuses unwanted," *Medical Ethics,* Vol. 5, No. 3 (1997), p. 95.

31. John F. Burns, "India Fights Abortion of Female Fetuses," *New York Times* (August 27, 1994), p. 5.

32. Madhu Kishwar, "Abortion of Female Fetuses: Is Legislation the Answer?" *Reproductive Health Matters,* Vol. 2 (1993), pp. 113–115.

7

International

Feminism

and

Reproductive

Rights

IF women are oppressed and suffer discrimination, as is clearly the case in India and probably also in China, can further restrictions on their reproductive freedom be justified? Is it reasonable to maintain that the idea of reproductive choice should apply only to women in Western countries because countries like China either refuse to recognize the concept of individual rights or claim that the need to control population growth overrides the value of leaving reproductive choices up to individuals?

The past decade has witnessed increasing calls worldwide for recognition of reproductive rights for all women, in whatever oppressive culture they may reside, and especially in those countries where governments or religious leaders have succeeded in curtailing reproductive rights. Efforts to ensure reproductive freedom for women, equal to that long enjoyed by men, would seem to further the interests of gender justice. But not according to the ideological stance of the feminists in India whose activism has led to legal prohibition of sex determination for the purpose of aborting female fetuses. According to this feminist group, women's reproductive right to abortion is subordinate to and even incompatible with gender justice. These Indian feminists focus on the class of women taken as a whole. Yet individual women suffer as much oppression, and their individual rights deserve as much protection. What is the "class of women" if not the sum of the individuals who are its members?

Women's reproductive rights remain intact if they are legally permitted to undergo prenatal diagnosis and subsequently choose to have an abortion if they discover that the sex of the fetus is female. Their reproductive rights are restricted if they are not allowed these options. One need not subscribe to the view that reproductive rights ought to be limitless or absolute to recognize that limiting the choices of Indian, Chinese, and other Asian women does restrict those rights. The ethical question is whether that limitation can be justified. I have argued that no one's rights are violated when laws permit sex determination, so limiting women's autonomy in this way appears to be unjustified. Perhaps the principle of beneficence can justify placing this limitation on reproductive freedom. But I cannot see how further restricting the options for women who already have limited choices in their lives can benefit them.

When I stated this position in the medical ethics journal published in

India, my article was attacked by one of the leaders of the Forum Against Sex-Determination and Sex-Preselection, the group that succeeded in enacting laws prohibiting sex determination. This is how she characterized my argument:

"Macklin's defense of SD [sex determination] in the name of 'women's right to privacy and liberty' reminds one of the Nazi murderers' 'right to privacy and liberty' to engineer genocide of the Jews in concentration camps located in remote places, away from the public eye. By this logic, every patriarch of the family has a right to abuse his wife and children in privacy of his home."[1] (In fact, my article referred to "reproductive rights" but did not specifically mention either a right to liberty or a right to privacy.) It is curious, to say the least, to find oneself compared with Nazi murderers for having argued that women in India and China deserve to have their reproductive rights respected.

One possibility is that the difference between my position, which defends reproductive liberty for women, and the Indian feminist's position, restricting liberty in the case of sex determination, stems from disparate cultural values. Our difference could then be explained by cultural relativism. But this is not a plausible explanation. What is relative here is not an ethical difference that derives from cultural diversity, but the difference between a particular strand of radical feminist ideology and the more dominant liberal feminist movement that emphasizes respect for the autonomy of women. My argument against laws prohibiting sex determination appeals to the same reproductive rights endorsed by women from countries throughout the world who attended the 1994 Cairo International Conference on Population and Development and the 1995 International Women's Conference in Beijing. The Indian feminist who criticized my published article calls this a "cold-blooded logic in the name of 'women's choice,' put forward in a social vacuum."[2] However, it was anything but a "social vacuum" that prompted me to undertake an ethical analysis of sex determination in India. A careful study of the plight of many women in that country, especially among the poorest classes, based on specific contextual facts, is what led me to assess the consequences for women of denying them the option to bear male children. Were it not for those grim consequences for women who do not have sons, it would be much easier to condemn the practice of aborting female fetuses as simply a prejudice against women and girl children.

In pointing out these grim consequences for Indian girls and women, I have been criticized as doing "a gutter inspector's job."[3] This accusation appears rooted in the same considerations that led the faculty and students at Wellesley College to question my right to speak about what goes on in India, a country and culture other than my own. It is also similar to the criticism by the Egyptian feminist of the white American male medical student who wrote about the health consequences of female genital mutilation in Africa—the resurrection of colonialism in "the white man's burden, medicalized."[4] It would be acceptable for an Indian woman to describe the plight of women and girls in India, but not for a North American. It is acceptable for African women to speak about the evils of female genital mutilation but not for American men, or for that matter, Western feminists. The curiosity in these cases is that the outsiders and their "insider" critics all agree on the substantive ethical content of the value judgments. The Indian feminist and I concur that gender discrimination does exist in India and is deplorable and that ways must be found to rectify injustices against women. The American medical student and the Egyptian feminist both oppose female genital mutilation as a harmful ritual practice. Yet those of us outside the cultures may not presume to describe the situation, much less criticize it from a "Western" perspective. This is "cultural sensitivity" taken to extremes. Were it sound, however, the Indian feminist would not be justified in her condemnation of Nazi murderers for engineering genocide of the Jews in concentration camps. Only Jews (or perhaps only non-Jewish Germans) could condemn the Nazis.

Can we meaningfully use the language of women's rights only when women have attained equal status and all forms of discrimination are abolished? Some defenders of cultural relativism argue that a call for recognition of rights is inappropriate in Asian countries and other parts of the world in which the values of individualism have not been parts of the traditional culture. This would deny to women in those regions significant rights in that sphere of life in which feminists in the West have fought so vigorously—human reproduction. Such a denial perpetuates global injustices.

The difference between the liberal and the radical brands of feminism is an ideological one that has nothing to do with the type of ethical relativism that stems from cultural diversity. The Indian feminist who criticized my article made that clear when she wrote: "We don't subscribe to the myopic world-view of the liberal school of thought which glorifies 'value-neutrality' and 'non-partisanship.'"[5] Although a vigorous defense of the right of women to exercise reproductive choices hardly seems to be "value neutral," the language of rights is a hallmark of liberal political thought. Those who would suppress the exercise of individual rights to attain what they consider "higher" values must, inevitably, believe they know what is best for all people or, in this case, all women. Either the idea of reproductive rights is a peculiarly Western value that should be limited to countries having a historical tradition of liberal political philosophy, or it rests on a universal moral principle that ought to be recognized everywhere in the world. The paternalism inherent in the radical feminist perspective that claims to know what is best for all diminishes women by denying their right to make choices for themselves.

Feminists Who Restrict Reproductive Rights

Like their arch conservative counterparts at the opposite extreme (on reproductive issues the religious right comes to mind), such feminists believe they know what is the morally right solution for everyone. I can think of no appropriate term in current use to refer to these feminists. Although *radical feminist* describes the viewpoint to which many members of this group subscribe, there may well be other radical feminists who do not. To claim to know what is best for others is accurately termed *paternalistic*, but all feminists, whatever their views, would no doubt recoil at being called *paternalist feminists*. I shall therefore refer to this group as *parentalist feminists* in the hope that, despite the infelicity of the term, it is as neutral a designation as is likely to be found.

On the one hand, parentalist feminists claim they are seeking to empower women. At the same time, they attempt to restrict the choices of women who already enjoy precious few options. Is it right for all Indian women to deny them by law the opportunity to choose the sex of their child? Is it right for all women to deny them the use of hormonal contraceptives and, beyond that, nonhormonal methods such as immunological contraceptives?

The rejection of hormonal methods by women's health activists in many countries follows international feminist groups such as FINRRAGE (Feminist International Network of Resistance to Reproductive and Genetic Engineering). These activists strongly oppose a variety of new reproductive technologies, both those that control fertility and those that seek to enhance it. FINRRAGE opposes techniques of assisted reproduction in general and in vitro fertilization in particular. The ideological premise underlying this position is that such technologies represent the newest effort by men to control women.

Several organized groups reject long-acting hormonal methods of contraception such as implants and injectables.[6] Their opposition to the introduction into family planning programs of the implant Norplant and the injectable Depo-Provera stems from the way these contraceptives work by altering the woman's natural hormonal system. The value that prompts their rejection is "adherence to nature." Hormonal methods "interfere with nature" in a way that barrier methods of contraception do not.

In India I met with a vocal feminist who espoused these views. Dr. Malini Karkal voiced adamant opposition to Norplant, the long-acting hormonal contraceptive. She said that the Population Council, a U.S. research organization that developed and is promoting the method, mentions in its literature "twelve problems with Norplant." Dr. Karkal expressed surprise that the Population Council is promoting it despite their acknowledgment of these 12 problems. I suggested that evidently the Population Council believes that the benefits of the method outweigh the risks so that despite the acknowledged 12 problems the method is sufficiently safe and effective to offer it as a choice to women. When Dr. Karkal still rejected the idea that Norplant could be acceptable, I asked for a more detailed explanation of her opposition.

Her answer made clear to me that the source of her opposition was rooted in international feminist ideology that follows the line propounded by FINRRAGE. Dr. Karkal replied that she is opposed to Norplant because "it is like genetic engineering. It's interfering in nature." Hormonal disturbances interfere with nature. Why should we encourage chemical, biological interferences with nature? She revealed this to be an aspect of her more general philosophy, which is opposed to the introduction of "unnatural" substances into the body.

The general claim that "what is unnatural is unethical" is an incoherent one in the modern, technological world. The particular application of the argument to hormonal methods of contraception rests on the perceived dangers of exogenous hormones. It is true that hormones have known side effects and may have long-term risks that are as yet unknown. But when one objects that scientific research has shown that the benefits, at least in most situations, outweigh the risks, the response from these opponents is that it is an article of faith to accept the premises and results of modern scientific inquiry, especially because the biomedical establishment is dominated by men, "techno-docs," who seek to control women.[7]

Dr. Karkal elaborated further on her objections to interfering with nature. Overall, she said, India has undergone modernization, industrialization, and Westernization. She indicted "Westernization" for focusing on technological fixes. An American doctor, she said, gives one pill to counteract another. It is a never-ending process of one technological remedy to counteract the bad effect of another. The views of this Indian feminist appear to be derived more from a branch of the international feminist movement than from contemporary cultural values in her own country. She attacks the values associated with Westernization, which might better be described as the values of modernity. Modern science and technology may well have had their roots in Western civilization, but Asian nations have by now embraced the technological aspects of modernity, for good or for ill.

It is surely true that preferences regarding methods of contraception vary according to culture, religion, ideology, and individual choice. However, women throughout the world have a deep desire to regulate their fertility. What vary from circumstance to circumstance and from individual to individual are the factors that influence their choice of contraceptives and whether women in some settings are even afforded a choice. The feminist groups who would deny women the choice of a long-acting, fertility-regulating drug insist that their value, opposition to hormonal methods, should rule for all women. One can respect the view that what is not natural is suspect and what is natural is better and still not seek to restrict women's right to informed choice. The key ethical requirement is that such choices must be well-informed and fully voluntary.

Some women do find the side effects of hormonal contraceptives intolerable. Maximizing choice for women would allow those who find hormonal methods unacceptable to use an alternative method of contraception. But many of the same feminist groups that oppose hormonal methods also oppose research and development of a potential long-acting, nonhormonal method: immunological contraceptives. In November 1993 the Women's Global Network for Reproductive Rights issued a call for an immediate halt to the development of immunological contraceptives. Their reasons for calling for an immediate halt to research on antifertility vaccines included the potential for abuse, manipulation of the immune system for contraceptive purposes without any benefits over existing methods, and past unethical clinical trials. The declaration was signed by 232 organizations from 18 different countries. By May 1996, the statement had been endorsed by 472 groups from 41 countries.[8]

Under "abuse potential," the document issued by this group asserts that "immunological contraceptives will not give women greater control over their fertility, but rather less." But the document fails to specify "less than what." The potential for abuse exists, as well, for other long-acting methods such as injectables and implants. This is one source of the Global Network's worry, and it cannot be dismissed because it is a legitimate cause for concern. Abuses of long-acting contraceptives in clinical research and in family planning programs have occurred over the years in several countries and were perhaps most serious in Brazil and India, the two countries with the largest number of signatories to the document issued by the Global Network. Their document rightly expresses concern about "mass administration of immunological contraceptives without people's knowledge or informed consent." Clearly, such practices violate the right of individuals to make reproductive choices. The question is whether the potential for abuse is so great that prohibition of antifertility vaccines is warranted and whether adequate safeguards might instead be put in place to guard against such abuse. Ironically, the possibility of developing additional nonhormonal methods is precluded by attempts to halt all research on an immunological method.

It is no doubt true that antifertility vaccines have the potential for abuse. But to say they have the *potential* for abuse is to imply that a potential also exists for appropriate ethical conduct of research and providing services. Those who would restrict women's options by limiting the range of contraceptive methods are, here again, being paternalistic in their attempt to curtail the freedom to choose. Just as the medical profession has long presumed to know what is best for women, now some women's health advocates hold a similar presumption. If antifertility vaccines can be shown to have a favorable benefit-risk ratio, as determined by women's own experiences as well as by scientific research, the ethically sound approach is not to foreclose those benefits but rather to combat the potential for abuse.

Another argument the Global Network makes is that "immunological contraceptives present no advantage for women over existing contraceptives." Yet that is precisely one of the questions research must seek to determine. If antifertility vaccines have fewer undesired side effects for women than hormonal methods, would that not be an advantage? If an immunological contraceptive is found to have only six problems, rather than the "twelve problems" of Norplant, would not the lesser number of problems be a benefit to women? Determining which contraceptives are more advantageous or beneficial than others is partly an objective, scientific question and partly a subjective judgment of the user. If one method is more efficacious than others in preventing pregnancy, that is an advantage. If one method has fewer unwanted side effects for users, that is also an advantage. An antifertility vaccine may be contraindicated for some people (those with a predisposition to allergies and autoimmune diseases), but so, too, are other contraceptive methods contraindicated for some people for different reasons. Of course, as the document states, "immunological contraceptives are unlikely to ever be harmless." But this is so for virtually every contraceptive method and for every medication. The ethical requirement is that the benefits to users must outweigh the risks of harm. Only well-designed, carefully conducted research can provide answers to questions about benefit-risk ratios.

The document asserts further that "human experimentation should only take place if the product being developed offers advantages over existing options. Immunological contraceptives offer no advantage. . . ." This conclusion begs the very question at issue in research: whether the investigational new drug offers greater advantages or poses fewer risks than existing methods. That question, too, can be properly answered only by carefully designed research that compares the immunological method with other available modes of contraception.

Some years after I first saw the document entitled "A Call for an Immediate Halt to Research on Antifertility Vaccines," I had the opportunity to meet with representatives of some of the feminist groups in Brazil that had signed onto the Global Network's statement.[9] One woman who heads a nongovernmental organization of women's health advocates in Recife, Brazil, said that her group had participated in the movement to stop work on the contraceptive vaccine. At a meeting of members of her nongovernmental organization and other women's health advocates, she argued that the vaccine represents a technological development based on a different principle from other contraceptives. It is based on the idea of immunization against pregnancy. This goes against the entire development of civilization, as a matter of principle.

Another point she and other opponents emphasized is that resources would be used for the vaccine and not for research and development of barrier methods. Long-term contraceptives are the leading methods in today's scientific and technological process. Most of the international resources are put into these methods, which are the ones physicians prefer, especially in developing countries. In sum, the woman from Recife argued, technology is not neutral. The very concept of "immunological contraception" is problematic. Another person at the conference followed up on those comments, stating that Brazilian women are very far removed from science and scientific knowledge. The position of Brazilian feminist groups opposed to the vaccine is close to the position of women generally in Brazil. It is thus a strategic point, related to the status and perceptions of women, as well as to the nature of a vaccine.

I found it difficult to grasp the argument that a contraceptive vaccine "by its very nature is different from a woman's individual desire." One participant said: "The concept of an immunological method against pregnancy is not an idea of women. It is a technology of science." It would seem to be true, on this line of reasoning, that any scientifically developed method of contraception is not "an idea of women." A monthly injection, a daily pill, or insertion of rods into the arm is not an idea that pops into the heads of people unfamiliar with modern methods of contraception.

The notion of an immunological method strikes Brazilian feminists and their counterparts elsewhere as significantly different from other scientifically developed methods. When I stated that feminist groups often presume to speak for uneducated and disadvantaged women, perhaps not always in the overall best interest of those women, one participant responded in this way. She noted that there are two currents in the Brazilian feminist movement. In one, individual feminists speak only for themselves. In the other, women speak for the group as a whole. This then leads to the problem of "representatives" in the feminist movement. What counts as true "representation" of women and their interests? A good question, one that deserves careful thought.

At another meeting in Brazil, held in Rio de Janeiro, one woman voiced a strong antitechnology ideology opposing all drugs that regulate fertility. Knowing what was likely to ensue, I asked her to elaborate on her opposition to research on immunological contraceptives. The first objection she cited was the fact that not much is known about the effects a contraceptive vaccine might have, and, in any case, it is not a "natural" substance to introduce into women's bodies. I replied that the very purpose of conducting research is to discover what effects it might have, to determine whether the potential benefits outweigh the risks, and to see whether this method might be more acceptable to women than hormonal methods and other currently available contraceptives. She said she was opposed to hormonal methods, too, and I remarked that this left women with relatively few choices.

The woman replied that barrier methods are the only acceptable contraceptives and that further research should be done in this area—a commonly held view among many feminists. Is it not possible, I asked, that using "barrier methods" (the various kinds are often lumped together) can place women at considerable risk of pregnancy and therefore, even greater risks to life and health should they decide to seek an abortion, since abortion in Brazil is illegal and typically unsafe? (It is important to keep in mind, however, that condoms—both male and female—are the only devices that provide reasonable protection against sexually transmitted diseases and HIV infection, surely an important consideration for women's health.)

At this point the speaker switched gears and introduced the familiar and overarching objection to research and development of immunological methods: the potential for abuse. I rehearsed the standard reply to this objection, asking whether efforts should not rather be focused on preventing such abuses, not only with regard to vaccines but also with other long-term contraceptive methods. However, as this particular feminist's position was opposed to all those other methods, as well, this strategy fell on deaf ears. She switched her argument once again: Too much money is being spent on this type of research and development, money that would be better spent on additional research on barrier methods and male methods. International funding agencies and pharmaceutical companies should devote resources to researching these other areas. However, this is not an all-or-nothing proposition. Research in all areas can and should go forward simultaneously. I pointed out that, ironically, a contraceptive vaccine could work just as well for men as for women.

When I asked my standard question about whether feminists are being paternalistic when they determine what is best for other women, this participant's reply was that she believes it is appropriate sometimes to choose for others. She cited the example of choices she makes for her children, an example that can almost always justify parentalistic actions. But, I asked, does she think women are like children in relevant respects? She did not reply to this challenge, but inquired whether my position is that it is never appropriate to limit people's choices. She cited the example of a hospital in Rio in which unsafe practices had been discovered. Activists chose to close the hospital (or the unsafe unit) down, and some women in the community objected because they said they were satisfied with the care they had been receiving. Was it wrong to decide for others, the participant asked, in order to protect women from unsafe conditions at the hospital they were happy with?

This is a good example of a circumstance in which people's "choices" may be justifiably limited because their choice was uninformed. The women may have experienced satisfaction as patients but were probably unaware that there were risks to themselves from unsafe practices. But this is where the analogy with the use of hormonal methods and immunological contraceptive development breaks down. There is widespread consensus among medically knowledgeable people throughout the world, as well as the women who use them, that hormonal contraceptives have a low enough level of risk to warrant their use. The purpose of immunological contraceptive research is to try to discover whether the same is true for that method. If vaccines turn out to have an unacceptably high level of risks they will not (or should not) be approved for use. To disapprove marketing of the product would be an instance of governmental paternalism—limiting women's options because the method is too unsafe to permit its use. Regulatory agencies, such as the Food and Drug Administration (FDA), do restrict the choices individuals might otherwise make and so can correctly be termed *paternalistic*. It is a "mixed" version of paternalism, however, because restrictions imposed by regulatory agencies can be justified on utilitarian grounds, as well. The paternalistic aspect is justifiable because ordinary citizens could not possibly determine on their own which drugs or devices are safe and effective.

What does all this have to do with ethical relativism? It would be nice to think that women throughout the world, in their common struggle against oppression, would emphasize the concerns that bind them together and work cooperatively to assert their autonomy, their liberty, and their collective power. Many women's groups do work toward that common goal in societies and cultures that differ from one another in many respects. But the branch of feminism that seeks to justify further limiting the choices of women whose reproductive options are already severely limited adheres to a rigid ideology regarding hormones and immunological vaccines. That stance rejects the distinctly different ethical premise of respect for autonomy, which grants to individuals the right decide what is most beneficial to themselves.

Does the parentalist ideology of this international group of feminists stem from a rejection of the Western value of individualism? Although the

Indian feminists I met with did not make this argument explicitly, it is one possible explanation for their unselfconscious denial that individual women should be permitted to choose what they believe is best for them. In contrast, the Brazilian feminists with whom I spoke strongly endorsed the idea of ensuring reproductive rights for women. They either did not notice, or did not care, that their endorsement of reproductive rights comes into direct conflict with their simultaneous rejection of making available hormonal or immunological contraceptives.

It would be a mistake, however, to think that all women's health advocates adopt the ideological position of the parentalist feminists, a position that grows out of a deep distrust of the male-dominated medical establishment. Some women's health advocates have shifted their initial position with the changing scientific developments and wider recognition by doctors and policy makers of women's perspectives on reproductive health. Anita Hardon, a long-standing participant in the women's health advocacy movement, was one of the authors of a book critical of the way Norplant was studied and introduced in several countries.[10] Along with other health advocates, Hardon began in 1989 to raise concerns about the safety of antifertility vaccines and about service delivery. Eight years later, Hardon questioned both the tactics and the unswerving position of the global network that continues to call for a halt to research and development of immunological contraceptives.[11] Hardon remains a champion of the user's perspective, arguing that the experience of women who use contraceptives may show that antifertility vaccines are more acceptable than hormonal methods. She has also questioned whether the women's health activists who continue in this campaign can claim that they represent the majority of potential users in an unbiased manner.

An ethical analysis that strives for universality can meaningfully ask whether reducing the options of women serves to benefit them as a class. Another meaningful question is whether women as individuals should be left free to decide for themselves what is in their own best interest. These questions are meaningful for those who adhere to the so-called liberal principles that mandate respect for persons and recognize as centrally important the rights and interests of individuals. They are not meaningful questions for those feminists who subscribe to a notion of "gender justice" that subordinates individual rights or who begin and end with opposition to what they consider male-dominated medical technology. That approach leaves little room for choices to be made by individual women. At the same time, we cannot ignore the long history of medical paternalism, which left women out of decision-making, or the coercive practices of population control carried out by many governments in developing countries over a 30-year period. In the 1990s, a shift occurred in the international arena from an emphasis on population control policies to that of promoting reproductive rights.

Feminists Who Promote Reproductive Rights

The parentalist feminists described above have sought to restrict women's reproductive rights in an attempt to protect them from perceived harms and abuses. In sharp contrast are women's health advocates throughout the world who are seeking to expand women's reproductive options and ensure their reproductive rights. In the matter of antifertility vaccines, many women's health advocates have adopted a different strategy from those calling for a halt to all research, focusing instead on safety, efficacy, and acceptability to women of this method.[12] A much broader effort demonstrated the nearly universal values shared by women in the work leading up to, during, and following the 1994 International Conference on Population and Development in Cairo (ICPD) and the 1995 International Women's Conference in Beijing. The consensus reached by a transnational coalition of women's rights and health advocates at the Cairo meeting included an application of basic human rights principles explicitly to governmental population policies and programs. Opposition to this view came from an alliance between the Catholic Church and Islamic religious fundamentalists, who contended that "reproductive rights" is a cover up for abortion rights, to which the Vatican remains unalterably opposed. It is not only abortion, however, but also contraception that the Vatican rejects, so its opposition to reproductive rights must be seen as encompassing all of what the women's groups at Cairo and Beijing sought to promote and ensure.

In a 3-week conference at the United Nations preparatory to the 1994 Cairo ICPD, the Vatican campaigned vigorously to exclude abortion from family planning services. Along with several countries including Honduras, Nicaragua, Malta, Benin, Morocco, Guatemala, and Argentina, the Vatican objected to wording in the United Nations plan such as the terms *reproductive health, reproductive rights, family planning,* and *safe motherhood.* The objection was based on the suspicion that those terms were "code words" sanctioning abortion.[13]

Women from many different countries who participated in the Cairo and Beijing conferences, and even more women who did not travel to those far-away cities, endorsed an ethical position that they claim is universal. Not only women but also a large number of men endorsed the Programme of Action of the ICPD. The broad ethical values embodied in the Programme of Action are equity, respect for human rights, application of human rights principles to population programs, rejection of coercion, violence, and discrimination, along with numerous more narrowly defined ethical values. To say that these values are universal is not to say that everyone in the world embraces them. Spokespersons for fundamentalist religions not limited to Roman Catholicism objected to the very language of "reproductive rights," as well as to numerous specific provisions endorsed by the Cairo consensus. Yet the fact that a consensus was reached in an international conference sponsored by the United Nations demonstrates that some fundamental ethical principles are recognized as universally valid and that most representatives from non-Western countries did not reject those principles as a form of Western cultural imperialism.

The wording of the general principles stated in the ICDP Programme of Action is the language of universality in ethics. A few examples of these principles are as follow:

> Principle 1: All human beings are born free and equal in dignity and rights. Everyone is entitled to all the rights and freedoms set forth in the Universal Declaration of Human Rights, without distinction of any kind, such as race, colour, sex, language, religion, political or other opinion, national or social origin, property, birth or other status. Everyone has the right to liberty and security of person.
> Principle 4: Advancing gender equality and equity and the empower-

ment of women, and the elimination of all kinds of violence against women, and ensuring women's ability to control their own fertility are cornerstones of population- and development-related programmes. The human rights of women and the girl child are an inalienable, integral and indivisible part of human rights. . . .

Principle 8: Everyone has the right to the enjoyment of the highest attainable standard of physical and mental health. . . . All couples and individuals have the basic right to decide freely and responsibly the number and spacing of their children and to have the information, education and means to do so.

What does it mean to claim universality for these (and other) principles? It is eminently clear what it does *not* mean. It does not mean that everyone in the world agrees with these principles, even at the very general level at which they are formulated. It does not mean that all who assent to the principles will always or even usually act in accordance with them. And it does not mean that even when people agree on the general formulations in which the principles are stated they will agree with specific attempts to apply the principles to concrete situations. So what good are such principles, and how can universality be claimed for them?

At the risk of stating the obvious or of being too simplistic, I have to go back to what normative ethics is all about. Ethics must be practical but it also has to embody ideals. Descriptive ethics is a factual account of how people actually behave. Normative ethics of necessity goes beyond what people actually do and states what they ought to do. Normative ethics should not be impossibly aspirational, but its very nature is to prescribe rather than to describe. If the principles adopted in the 1994 ICPD seem to go well beyond what people and governments actually do, it does not show that the principles themselves are not universal. It is simply a reminder that the actual behavior of individuals, groups, and government often falls short of the ethical principles they espouse.

Yet representatives of some governments, along with the Vatican, objected vigorously to many of the statements in drafts leading up to the final document. A month before the Cairo conference was to begin, the Vatican sent envoys to Islamic countries seeking allies in opposition to the draft document. The Vatican denied that it was looking for an alliance only with Islamic leaders, contending that it appealed to leaders of all religions against what it viewed as an attack on the family and traditional sexual morality. The government of Iran backed the Vatican's position on the draft document, as did that of Libya. Leaders at Al Azhar Islamic University in Cairo, a prestigious center of Islamic education, denounced the draft ICPD document as offensive to Islam in language similar to that of the Vatican, although the statement from Al Azhar did not mention the Vatican.[15]

Once the conference began, the Vatican strengthened its opposition to the draft document, rejecting various compromises offered by other delegates. On September 6, Vatican diplomats blocked a consensus on a formula that was sponsored by Pakistan, an Islamic nation. The compromise formula was also supported by Benin, formerly a Vatican ally, as well as by Iran.[16] In the end, the Vatican dropped its opposition to a controversial paragraph on abortion that had occupied days of debate by the delegates. In what was already a compromise, the draft paragraph referred to "the health impact of unsafe abortion," to which the Vatican objected on the grounds that there is no such thing as a "safe" abortion because it involves the death of a human being. The Vatican's efforts were bent on eliminating all language that might suggest that abortion was a right of women.[17] The final draft paragraph (8.25) stated:

> In no case should abortion be promoted as a method of family planning. All Governments and relevant intergovernmental and nongovernmental organizations are urged to strengthen their commitment to women's health, to deal with the health impact of unsafe abortion as a major public health concern and to reduce the recourse to abortion through expanded and improved family-planning services. . . ."

In the end, delegates from the Vatican and from some Islamic countries said they were still uncomfortable with some of the wording in the document. Delegates from several Muslim nations said they did not approve of the way the document called for reproductive rights for individuals rather than couples.[18] Despite the views of these and other official delegates to the United Nations conference, women in Catholic and Islamic countries openly disagree, and their actions in seeking abortions and using birth control are in direct defiance of what religious and political leaders in their countries proclaim.

How do all these events bear on the debate about cultural and ethical relativism and the charge of ethical imperialism on the part of Western nations? Let us begin with the Pope. In his unrelenting attack on women's choice to use contraceptives or undergo abortions, Pope John Paul II took the position that Western feminist cultural imperialists were responsible for influencing people in non-Western cultures to adopt their views. In a conversation with Nafis Sadik, the executive director of the United Nations Population Fund, the Pope implied that she was a dupe of Western feminist cultural imperialism. Sadik, a Pakistani Muslim, spearheaded the 1994 Cairo conference and was among the world leaders calling for recognition of the reproductive rights of women.[19] A report of a remarkable interview said that the Pope found Sadik's position to be the product of American feminism, a form of "destructive cultural imperialism."[20] When Sadik asked the Pope how many Catholics he thought actually follow the teachings of the Catholic church in the matter of contraception and abortion, he replied "It's only the Catholics in those materialistic developed societies who don't. All the people in the poorer countries do."[21] The Pope opined further that in Western societies the family is disintegrating and ethical values are gone. Observing that the Pope's use of his power and authority is the essence of imperialism, one commentator on the conversation between Sadik and the Pope asks: "Who's the cultural imperialist?"[22]

It is a fallacy to argue that because reproductive rights were first recognized and established in Western nations, the expansion of those concepts to non-Western cultures is a form of cultural imperialism. The needs of women in all parts of the globe are similar, although the social and cultural contexts vary considerably. Women everywhere have suffered the consequences of unwanted pregnancy, of having too many children, or of bearing children when they are too young or too old to safely undergo pregnancy and childbirth. The devastating health consequences of lack of access to contraceptives and safe, legal abortion are universal, crossing boundaries of nations and cultures and religions. For decades these concerns were largely addressed using the language of health. For the first time, the 1994 Cairo ICPD conference shifted the terminology to the language of rights.

Women's rights activists worked together in an international alliance in the years preceding the Cairo conference. Women's nongovernmental organizations in Asia, Africa, and the Middle East, as well as in North and South America, embraced the language of rights as pertaining to reproduction and sexuality as well as to other areas of social and political life. This worldwide alliance and collaboration among women's groups does not mean that all women everywhere have identical values and subscribe to exactly the same exceptionless moral rules. It does mean, however, that women everywhere recognize restrictions on their reproductive choices to be discriminatory, whether those restrictions are imposed by the government, by religious authorities, or by their own husbands.

The use of rights language has political as well as ethical implications. As Rosalind Petchesky observes, the shift from a health perspective to a reproductive rights perspective in the United Nations conference arose out of the felt need of women's movements everywhere to state a strong response to the rising tide of conservatism and religious fundamentalism.[23] Rights language offers a more likely prospect of achieving political gains than does the language of health, as important as the latter remains for setting medical and health policies. Especially in democratic countries, but increasingly in all parts of the world, the charge that rights are being violated gets people's attention. With the exception of a few countries that remain authoritarian holdouts in a community of nations that at least pays lip service to democracy, it is unpopular, if not entirely unacceptable, to maintain that women's rights count for less than those of men. And it is women's rights that the Cairo Programme articulated in its statements regarding reproductive health and sexuality.

An entire chapter of the 1994 ICPD Programme of Action is devoted to "Gender Equality, Equity and Empowerment of Women." These developments could not have occurred without the cooperation of and endorsement by men in positions of power and authority throughout the world. Thus while it is true that the reproductive and sexual rights articulated in the Cairo document are not accepted or agreed to by every individual on the planet, that does not make these values any the less universal. The denial by the Vatican and fundamentalist religious leaders that such rights ought to be recognized hardly constitutes a denial of the validity of the rights claims. Slaveholders in the antebellum South denied that blacks had a right to be free, Hitler denied that Jews, gypsies, and homosexuals had a right to reside in Germany, and the Nazi regime ultimately rejected their right to life. The denial of rights claims by traditional authorities and those who wield power have little to do with the universality of ethical principles and everything to do with adherence to religious ideology and political might.

The United Nations–sponsored international conferences in Cairo and Beijing brought together women from North and South, East and West, developed and developing countries. Cultural, ethnic, and religious differences among the women tended to be subordinated to their common concerns and a common agenda: recognition of women's rights, including reproductive rights, women's social and political equality, and their struggle against oppression and discrimination. With a practical agenda rooted in real-world concerns, these conferences virtually obliterate the theoretical differences that tend to divide academic feminists.

Despite the underlying truth of the slogan "sisterhood is global," a striking difference is apparent between feminists in developing countries and the activities of most academic feminists in the United States. The U.S. feminist literature is rife with disagreements about highly theoretical matters, for example, whether feminism should embody an "ethics of care?" Some critics argue that emphasis on caring and nurturance merely perpetuates the subordinate role of women as caregivers, helpmeets, and family members responsible for care and nurture. A different debate begins by asking: Is an approach that emphasizes women's political, economic, educational, and social rights the proper way to go about correcting ongoing injustices to women? One strand of feminist theory contends that an emphasis on autonomy, rights, and justice is just another way of buying into "masculine" concepts. This latter theoretical perspective divides the concepts into the categories of "masculine" and "feminine," locating rights and justice in the masculine sphere.

Feminists from several developing countries harshly criticized an educational seminar on feminist theory held at an American university.

The international participants (eight women and two men) came from Mexico, Uruguay, Brazil, India, South Africa, the Philippines, and China. In a post-seminar, day-long meeting that I was invited to facilitate, they were amazed at the bickering among American theorists of feminism and appalled that the conference contained little, if any, discussion of practical and political concerns that constitute the main agenda in their own countries. It is true that many of these international participants were activists rather than academics, and speakers at the seminar were all from the ivory tower. Still, the participants deplored the lack of concrete application of "abstract" feminist theory to the real issues they confront in the struggle for women's reproductive rights and equality in their countries.

One international participant from South Africa later wrote: "My overall impression was how different and on the move things are back here. . . . Many of our deliberations were around airy academic issues — and I had thought ethics was about ensuring that those who are most vulnerable are protected; that people who are poor or part of minority groups are afforded protection by the dominant patriarchal biomedical establishment."[24]

On an encouraging note, several leading feminist scholars in the United States who work in the field of bioethics have sought to emphasize themes shared by different feminist schools of thought, trying to unite rather than further divide what has become a fragmented women's movement elevated to an atmospheric level of theory. Karen Rothenberg, a lawyer-ethicist, uses the themes shared by feminist theories to enrich the analysis of a public policy issue unrelated to reproductive issues: the Maryland Health Care Decisions Act, which addresses the need for a comprehensive legislative approach to end-of-life decisions.[25] Susan Sherwin acknowledges the evident truth that "contemporary feminism cannot be reduced to a single, comprehensive, totalizing theory" and strives in her work to use the minimal number of theoretical commitments.[26] Rosemarie Tong makes explicit a call for feminist theorists to come together: "Like the time for unity without diversity, the time for diversity without unity is past. We feminist bioethicists need to achieve 'unity-in-diversity.'"[27]

As detached as academic feminist theory has been from many of the concerns addressed by nongovernmental, activist women's groups in developing countries, a more ominous threat looms. That is the tendency to challenge the concept of ethical universality from the perspective of postmodern multiculturalism, which threatens the very cause feminists have sought to promote. As one writer notes: "Ironically, the Western feminist, postmodernist critique of modernity in the name of cultural diversity could increase many women's vulnerability to right-wing male exploitation . . . on behalf of premodern patriarchal norms."[28]

Postmodern feminism rejects the underlying assumptions of other branches of feminist thought. As in postmodernism generally, postmodern feminism denies the existence of an objective reality that can describe the "essential" woman.[29] This approach is "to consider real life experiences influenced by each woman's race, class, age, and sexual orientation."[30] In effect, every option is left open. Once we "consider" the particular "situated" realities of all individual women, on what basis can ethical judgments be made? After due "consideration," how should we act?

If this postmodern version of feminism evokes memories of the approach known as *situation ethics* promoted in the early years of bioethics, it has even worse consequences. Joseph Fletcher, the chief spokesperson for situation ethics, called for decision-makers in medical matters to explore all facets of each situation to arrive at a "loving and humane solution." Fletcher opposed a dogmatic, rule-oriented approach to ethics but had few doubts about which were the "right" ethical standards to embrace. Postmodernism—in its feminist guise or more generally—is equally situational but denies that there are any "right" ethical standards to embrace.

Notes

1. Vibhuti Patel, "The Ethics of Gender Justice," *Medical Ethics*, Vol. 3, No. 4 (1995), p. 65.

2. Patel, p. 65.

3. Patel, p. 66.

4. Soheir Morsy, "Safeguarding Women's Bodies: The White Man's Burden Medicalized," *Medical Anthropological Quarterly*, Vol. 5, No. 1 (1991), p. 19–23.

5. Patel, 65.

6. See, for example, Barbara Mintzes, Anita Hardon, and Jannemieke Hanhart (eds.), *Norplant: Under Her Skin* (Amsterdam: Eburon, Women's Health Action Foundation, 1993).

7. The term *techno-docs* is used by Patel, p. 65. I first came across it in an article by the radical feminist Gena Corea, who says that the term was conceived by the head of the Yale University in vitro fertilization team to describe himself and his colleagues. Since then, the term has been transformed into a pejorative one by feminists who follow the FINRRAGE persuasion. Gena Corea, "Junk Liberty," (ed.) Larry Gostin, *Surrogate Motherhood: Politics and Privacy* (Bloomington: Indiana University Press, 1988), p. 334, n. 2.

8. Anita Hardon, "Contesting Claims on the Safety and Acceptability of Anti-Fertility Vaccines," *Reproductive Health Matters*, No. 10 (1997), pp. 68–81.

9. The visit to Brazil in April 1996 was part of my second Ford Foundation project on ethics and reproductive health.

10. Mintzes, Hardon, and Hanhart (eds.), *Norplant: Under Her Skin.*

11. Hardon, pp. 76–78.

12. Hardon, p. 76.

13. Susan Chira, "Abortion Is Divisive Issue at Population Talks," *New York Times* (April 24, 1994), p. 18.

14. Programme of Action of the United Nations International Conference on Population and Development, ICPD Secretariat, U.N. Doc. A/CONF.171/13 (1994).

15. John Tagliabue, "Vatican Seeks Islamic Allies in UN Population Dispute," *New York Times* (August 18, 1994), pp. A1, A8.

16. Alan Cowell, "Vatican Rejects Compromise on Abortion at UN Meeting," *New York Times* (September 7, 1994), pp. A1, A8.

17. Barbara Crossette, "Vatican Drops Fight Against UN Population Document," *New York Times* (September 10, 1994), p. 5.

18. Chris Hedges, "Key Panel at Cairo Talks Agrees on Population Plan," *New York Times* (September 13, 1994), p. A10.

19. Lisa M. Hisel, "Who's the Cultural Imperialist?" Editorial page (no number), and Carl Bernstein and Marco Politi, "The Angry Pope," *Conscience*, Vol. XVII, No. 4 (Winter 1996–97), pp. 14–17.

20. Bernstein and Politi, p. 17.

21. Bernstein and Politi, p. 17.

22. Hisel, "Who's the Cultural Imperialist?"

23. Rosalind Pollack Petchesky, "From Population Control to Reproductive Rights: Feminist Fault Lines," *Reproductive Health Matters*, No. 6 (November 1995), pp. 152–161.

24. Marion Stevens, "The Feminist Bioethics Course," *IN/FIRE Ethics*, Vol. 4, No. 2/3 (1995), p. 2.

25. Karen H. Rothenberg, "Feminism, Law, and Bioethics," *Kennedy Institute of Ethics Journal*, Vol. 6, No. 1 (1996), pp. 69–84.

26. Susan Sherwin, *No Longer Patient* (Philadelphia: Temple University Press, 1992), p. 32.

27. Tong, p. 51.

28. Rosemary Radford Ruether, "Women and Culture," *Conscience*, Vol. XVI, No. 4 (Winter 1995–96), p. 15.

29. Rothenberg, p. 74.

30. Rothenberg, p. 74.

8

International Research and Ethical Imperialism

DESPITE the postmodern claim that there are no objectively right ethical standards, hardly anyone denies that ethically right standards must govern biomedical research involving human subjects. Yet the international research enterprise gives rise to many of the same debates surrounding cultural and ethical relativism as we have seen in other biomedical arenas. A prominent view holds that research involving human subjects must embody ethical universals rather than be tailored to the norms and practices of particular cultures. One expression of the universal view states: "If it is unethical to carry out a type of research in a developed country, it is unethical to do that same research in a developing country." This requirement for uniformity seeks to ensure that justice prevails in the conduct of research that crosses national boundaries. It is also designed to protect vulnerable populations from exploitation. An underlying assumption of this "protectionist" stance is that people in developing countries are somehow vulnerable to exploitation in a way that people in developed countries are not. That assumption bears examination and is open to challenge as developing country researchers and ministries of health have begun to acquire the capacity for scientific and ethical review similar to what is already established in developed countries.

A different view—we may call it "ethical pluralism"—holds that rules governing research practices may vary according to the cultural norms accepted in the country where the research is carried out. "Respect for diversity" underlies the approach of ethical pluralism, which rejects the idea that a single set of ethical standards for research should prevail in our culturally diverse world.

The United States has elaborate and detailed federal regulations governing biomedical and behavioral research, whereas many countries in the world have no such laws, regulations, or procedures for protecting human subjects, and others have only the barest minimum. Conflicts are bound to arise in international collaborative research where a country in which research is being carried out lacks the norms or mechanisms that have become accepted standards by the sponsoring agency. If researchers in those countries must adhere to regulations promulgated by the U.S. government, some people object that it is a form of "ethical imperialism." But if researchers in some countries need not be bound by ethical standards widely accepted in the conduct of research, it would appear to validate ethical relativism.

Differences among cultures—especially with regard to the primacy of the individual—have led some people to argue that informed consent is a concept understandable and applicable in the West but is irrelevant to social and cultural norms in Africa and Asia. For example, at a conference sponsored by the World Health Organization in December 1980, the World Health Organization's Proposed International Ethical Guidelines for Human Experimentation were first presented. One conference participant from the United States described the guidelines as "essentially based on American standards of ethical review as well as on the international codes"—the Nuremberg Code and the Declaration of Helsinki.[1] This concern was also voiced by some participants from developing countries at the conference, who objected to elements of the proposed guidelines on grounds of ethical imperialism: "How far, they wondered, can Western countries impose a certain concept of human rights? In countries where the common law heritage of individuality, freedom of choice, and human rights do not exist, the . . . guidelines may seem entirely inappropriate."[2]

Interestingly, just the opposite worry has been voiced by individuals from developing countries. In recent decades and even today, some research has been carried out in developing countries that cannot be conducted in North America and Western Europe. Critics of a "double standard" from both the West and from developing countries argue that if a research project is deemed ethically questionable or unethical in a developed country it ought not to be conducted in a developing country, especially one that lacks a process for research review. Even where there does exist a mechanism for ethical review of research in a developing country, the norms of that country might not recognize as wide an array of individual rights as is common in the West, so ethical review committees could find it perfectly acceptable to proceed with a research design that would not be approved in North America or Europe. It is at least an apparent contradiction to seek to have it both ways, arguing on the one hand that research considered unethical in the United States should not be conducted in Africa or Asia, and at the same time contending that ethical values vary from one place to another so it is ethical imperialism to impose Western values on non-Western cultures.

Although the "contradiction" related to ethical imperialism may be implicit and is more of an inconsistency than a strict logical contradiction, it has its roots in past episodes of exploitation. For example, a study was carried out in the 1950s on poor Puerto Rican women during the initial phases of testing the effectiveness of the pill as a contraceptive. The ethical basis on which this study was faulted was the absence of the subjects' informed consent,[3] and it is clear that researchers would not have done the study on the U.S. mainland without informing women that they were involved in a research project or about the side effects they might experience, including the chance of becoming pregnant.[4] At the time the study was conducted there were as yet no federal regulations and no federally mandated institutional review boards in this country. So even though it would not have violated laws or regulations to carry out this type of study without properly informing women, it is evident that the scruples of researchers prevented their doing the same study on more educated women in the United States.

The research that used poor women in Puerto Rico as subjects highlights the need to distinguish between an explanation of an event and an ethical justification. One writer surmises that the most compelling reason for choosing this subject population was convenience: "Lower income groups were more available for this type of mass experimentation . . . and were less likely than well-heeled mainlanders to mount political protests or initiate lawsuits."[5] A more cynical supposition is that "perhaps there was also a latent racism at work."[6] Neither proposed explanation could possibly provide an ethical justification. Critics have rightly contended that what occurred was exploitation: conducting research in other countries that could not, for ethical reasons, be carried out in the United States.

Nevertheless, when required by international sponsors to employ rigorous procedures to obtain voluntary, informed consent from subjects, some researchers in non-Western countries have complained that it is "ethical imperialism" to impose North American procedures requiring strict adherence to informed consent on cultures in which patients normally do not have to give consent to treatment or research maneuvers.

Several years ago I was a member of a group assembled by the Centers for Disease Control and Prevention (CDC) to discuss a number of ethical issues that arose in a proposed collaborative study between the CDC and medical researchers in China. The study was to take place in a rural area where there was a high incidence of birth defects. The study design involved the use of a placebo for some participants, while others would receive a substance that researchers thought might reduce the likelihood of birth defects. The Chinese collaborator was resisting the ethical requirement of obtaining individual informed consent from prospective subjects. Some CDC officials thought that the Chinese researcher's objections were valid, given the differences in biomedical research and practice in the United States and the People's Republic of China. Our standards of informed consent to treatment seem rarely to apply in China, and up to that time there had been relatively few clinical trials similar to those common in the United States and Europe.

The Chinese physician stated his opposition to the informed consent requirement on two separate grounds. First, obtaining consent from patients is an altogether alien idea in medical practice, so to introduce it into the research context would be unfamiliar to many Chinese participants and likely to arouse suspicion. A population unacquainted with biomedical research would have difficulty understanding why physicians would seek their permission to do something because doctors normally do what they believe is best for patients without the need to ask. Second, the Chinese physician argued, if potential subjects were told that half would get placebo, no one would enroll because the concept of a placebo (or, at least, a placebo-controlled study) is unheard of in China. If people knew there was a possibility that they would get a dummy pill instead of an active substance no one would agree to participate and so, he argued, whatever information they are given should not include mention of the placebo control. In addition to the two main reasons the researcher stated, an additional complication is the Chinese cultural tradition of involving the family and even the larger community in individual health-related matters. In sum, the researcher said that if the CDC required the informed consent of Chinese participants, it would be impossible for him to carry out the study.

Some CDC officials questioned whether it would constitute ethical imperialism to impose on China researchers requirements drawn from U.S. regulations. Several of us at the meeting argued that it was not specific U.S. government regulations that were being imposed, but rather worldwide principles articulated in documents such as the Declaration of Helsinki, an international statement first adopted in 1964 by the World Medical Association and amended several times since then at periodic meetings of the World Medical Assembly.

After much discussion, the group reached a consensus that the use of placebos in research would be unethical if subjects are not informed that they will either receive active medication or placebo. The discussion was complicated by the literal translation of *placebo* offered by the Chinese researcher. He gave a Chinese translation of the phrase "makes people comfortable," which accurately conveys the meaning of *placebo* in the treatment setting but is misleading in the context of research. The group insisted that he use different Chinese words that would convey the true meaning of *placebo* in the research setting.

Several years after that meeting at the CDC, I learned what the Chinese researcher had actually done. The physician who was the principal investigator attended a conference in the United States and described the cultural compromise he and his collaborators had reached.[7] He reiterated his belief that no one would agree to join the study if the researchers sought consent only from the individual women who were potential subjects. In Chinese culture women have to involve their husbands, their family, and their community leaders. The researchers developed a process of "community consent," which involved different levels of the community, at the county, township, and village levels. All had to agree for subjects to be enrolled. Researchers spoke with government leaders at every level. Next, they talked to the health authorities at each level. Professional people from all these levels also had to understand and approve the research. Then, finally, there was the family. The entire family then had to approve, but the actual role of the family depended on who was the head. The physician would tell the woman "it is good for health reasons" for her to take the pill. After this whole process was completed, the woman came to the physician/researcher, who explained everything to her. The physician, not the woman, signed the consent form. It took about 3 months for all these steps to be accomplished.

Although the procedures differed considerably from those typically employed in Western countries, the solution the researchers arrived at sought to adapt the Western requirement of obtaining informed consent from the individual to the family- and community-oriented situation in China. While the women participants in the study appeared to be reasonably well informed, they alone did not consent to participate in the study. One aspect of the procedure that would not be acceptable to most research ethics committees in the United States is the physician's statement that "for health reasons, it is good for the woman to take the pill." That could not truthfully be claimed (at least, not in advance) for those women who received a placebo instead of the study medication, nor could positive health benefits be guaranteed for the experimental drug. The researcher maintained that in the absence of some such statement, no one would consent to participate and the study could not be carried out.

It is critically important to distinguish between the specific procedures embodied in U.S. regulations and the fundamental principle demanding that we respect as individuals the persons who are enlisted as subjects of research. Respect for persons is properly understood as the ethical principle designed to protect the rights of human subjects of biomedical and behavioral research, in particular, the right to self-determination. The reason why informed consent is an ethical requirement even when the proposed research carries a very low or virtually nonexistent risk of harm, as in some social or behavioral investigations, is that people can be wronged even when they are not harmed. To carry out perfectly benign studies on human beings without their knowledge or consent would wrong them because their right to self-determination is violated. In the absence of their granting voluntary, informed consent, research subjects would be treated as a mere means to the ends of others, as objects or instruments rather than as persons worthy of respect.

But what about cultures in which individuals are not granted the right of self-determination in other areas of life? It is just this focus on the individual that is criticized as uniquely American or, at least, Western. Lisa Newton, a philosopher from the United States, argued that "[i]t is 'ethical imperialism' at its worst to assume that the informed consent requirement, which does indeed serve one (only one) moral principle in the Western setting, is in itself such a universal ethical standard."[8] Newton contends that there is today a growing doubt surrounding the value of individualism and individual rights, so "the investigator might better stick to the research and accept the local assessment as to adequate protection of individual rights."

Exactly the opposite position is stated by another American bioethicist, Ruth Faden, and co-author Carel B. Ijsselmuiden, a physician from South Africa, who write: "Appeals to cultural sensitivity . . . are no substitute for careful moral analysis. We see no convincing arguments for a general policy of dispensing with, or substantially modifying, the researcher's obligation to obtain first-person consent in biomedical research conducted in Africa." Interestingly, Ijsselmuiden and Faden add that defenders of such a policy "have relied on limited and often dated anthropologic literature that does not reflect the rapid cultural changes brought about by colonialism and independence, warfare, and urbanization."[9]

The danger of a reliance solely on local assessment is that in societies where there is no tradition whatsoever of individual rights, the local assessment may reject the very concept that individual research subjects have rights, and therefore they may be enrolled simply with the permission of the village chief. Even if it is the custom for a village chief to decide what everyone in that village is permitted or required to do in the ordinary activities of the village, it does not follow that the chief should be granted the same authority to submit members of his village to research maneuvers at the hands of biomedical or social scientists. Lisa Newton's observation that there is today a growing doubt surrounding the value of individualism and individual rights may well be accurate, but that doubt exists mainly in the minds of academics who live comfortable lives in a nation whose Bill of Rights stands as a bedrock of constitutional democracy. No corresponding doubts are to be found among advocates of democratic reform in China or in the many Latin American countries in which dictators reigned until very recently. In countries whose members struggle against dictators or oppression at the hands of autocratic rulers, reformers strive for recognition of individual rights.

The conduct of international collaborative research requires ongoing attention to these concerns. In one instance, a research proposal from an

African country designed to study fertility awareness and pregnancy avoidance stated that "village chiefs will also assure the women of the need to cooperate." The program officer from the international agency to which the proposal was submitted wrote back to the principal investigator: "This implies pressure from the village chiefs, and also implies that the women who participate in the study will be known to them." The program officer's letter added: "you state 'the consent that we anticipate is almost taken for granted in our own part of the country.' Again, as you well understand, consent should be informed and entirely voluntary." In his reply, the principal investigator expressed his knowledge of and willingness to comply with these ethical requirements. The researcher's letter said:

> In Nigeria, there is no ethical problem in dealing with human subjects relating to information gathering. The intensity of research activities in various parts of Nigeria also reveals that Nigerian women are more than willing to answer questions relating to their sexuality. . . . [E]merging new experiences corrected the earlier insinuations that Nigerian rural women might be unwilling to discuss what might be regarded as private affairs.
>
> In the present circumstance, the village chiefs are routinely informed of any project to be executed in their villages as part of courtesy to them as the head of the village and for him to be in the know of things going on around him. He, in any case, does not know the individual women to be interviewed. In our case, we do not anticipate any ethical problem on this: indeed the consent of the village chief is taken for granted because it is freely and willingly given. The responses to questions from women are to be held confidential. Those unwilling to be interviewed are normally not coerced to respond. Therefore the issue of pressure does not arise at all.[10]

It is evident that the Nigerian researcher was well aware of the ethical requirements of the sponsoring agency and sought to assure the sponsor that the ethical precepts of voluntariness of participation and preserving confidentiality would be adhered to. What happened in the actual conduct of the research is, of course, impossible to know.

There are, to be sure, instances of bureaucratic foolishness in international collaborative research when researchers mindlessly apply procedural rules. A researcher from the United States was doing a study in Bangladesh for which he was required by his home institution's research ethics committee to use their standard consent form.[11] On the boilerplate portion of the form, the instructions stated that in case of any questions or problems about the research, subjects should call the research office of the university in the United States (collect). The sponsoring institution's insistence on using its standard consent form is an example of a procedure that is utterly meaningless and irrelevant to ensuring the ethics of research carried out in Bangladesh.

Other requirements would not deserve the label "bureaucratic foolishness," but are nevertheless procedural requirements rather than principled ethical standards. A member of an ethical review committee from New Zealand wrote that no approval by an institutional review board from the United States that he knew of would be valid in his country. That is because the U.S. institutional review boards do not meet the requirements for accreditation in New Zealand. In that country, research ethics committees must have equal numbers of lay (community) and professional members; decisions of the committee must be made by consensus, not majority vote; and two of the members must be representatives of local Maori tribes. Institutional review boards in the United States must have at least one community member; there are no rules for how a committee must reach its decisions and no requirements for inclusion of members of specific groups. The New Zealand requirements rely on certain assumptions about how best to arrive at ethical decisions in the area of biomedical research: Medical professionals should not dominate in the approval process, a simple majority vote could approve a research protocol by too slim a margin to be ethically acceptable, and minority groups should be well represented. Valid though they may be in guaranteeing a fair process of decision-making, these requirements do not count as substantive ethical standards but are best seen as procedural safeguards. However, it is often hard to make a sharp distinction between procedural requirements and substantive ethical standards, because the point of some procedural safeguards is to ensure fairness, a matter of ethical principle.

Spousal Authorization for Research

At a meeting I attended in Bangladesh, participants defended the practice of obtaining spousal authorization for women's enrollment in research.

The prevailing cultural practice in Bangladesh is to obtain a husband's "consent" for his wife's use of contraceptives and for her participation in research. I offered the unqualified claim that women should be treated as independent adults and that a cultural practice that prevails in other social contexts is not ethically acceptable in the research enterprise. This position was greeted with skepticism, if not outright rejection, by many participants in the meeting. I defended my view with the observation that biomedical and social research have by now become an international enterprise, with established standards of ethical practice. One such standard is respect for the autonomy of research subjects and protection of their confidentiality, even with regard to members of their own family.

A similar discussion took place at a meeting in Nigeria, in which participants insisted they could not carry out their research at all without first obtaining the husband's consent to involve his wife. This creates the dilemma of whether researchers may employ a practice that would violate an ethical standard of the sponsoring country or agency and proceed with the research, or whether they should forgo doing the research and thereby lose the opportunity to learn information that is critically important for improving the condition of women in their country. What was not explored in that discussion was precisely what would happen if the researchers sought to go forward and recruit the women without first obtaining permission from their husbands. Would the women refuse to be subjects? If they did agree to participate but did not want their husbands to know, how would their husbands discover that their wives were participants in the research? Was this simply a case of researchers adhering to a social practice because of the existence of the social norm? Might they seek to circumvent that norm and thereby succeed in doing the research without violating the ethical requirement to preserve the confidentiality of research participants? These questions were not addressed, but it would be useful to know the answers in order to learn what would be the consequences of failing to adhere to that cultural norm.

One journal article described a workshop on research ethics in Uganda that addressed the problem of acquiescence by another family member for an individual to participate in research.[12] The Ugandan setting appears to be similar to the research in China described earlier, where not only the husband but also other groups had to be consulted before individual subjects could be enrolled. In Uganda, however, the situation was further complicated by the simultaneous existence of customary or traditional practices and modern, civil law. The latter states that an 18-year-old male living at home has the legal right to make his own decision. But customary law dictates that the son must first obtain his father's permission. Ugandan women are even further restricted by the need to obtain the permission of their partner before they may agree to serve as a research subject.

Participants in the Ugandan workshop arrived at a compromise solution between the conflicting demands of customary law and the principle of respect for autonomy as it applies to research. The group recommended a 48-hour waiting period between the time researchers solicit subjects' participation and the time they sign a consent form. During that period, subjects may confer with family members, if they wish, before deciding finally whether to participate. A family member could ask the researcher questions about the research that might arise in the course of a family discussion. The workshop group agreed, however, that another family member could not offer an individual as a research subject if that person was unwilling. The Ugandan group did not view the concept of autonomy as entirely alien to their culture when applied to the research context. Instead, they arrived at a compromise not unlike the one fashioned by the Chinese researcher who collaborated with the CDC. It thus seems possible to respect the autonomy of the individual and at the same time respect the cultural practice of involving the family.

Nevertheless, a strict requirement that a husband must first grant permission before researchers may enroll his wife in research does violate the "respect for persons" ethical principle. That principle mandates equal respect to women as persons. The requirement of spousal authorization for a woman's participation in research was addressed by a panel of the Special Programme of Research, Development, and Research Training in Human Reproduction (HRP) of the World Health Organization. This panel, the Scientific and Ethical Review Group, developed a document entitled *Guidelines on Reproductive Health Research and Partners' Agreement*, which was subsequently approved and disseminated by the HRP program officials.

The guidelines state that "a requirement of partner agreement or authorization for an individual to participate in research violates the autonomy of research subjects and their right to confidentiality. Therefore, as a matter of ethical principle, a requirement of partner agreement or authorization should not be permitted in studies supported by the Special Programme. . . ."[13] However, the guidelines also note that it is "because of existing cultural, religious, political or legal constraints, it is sometimes impossible to achieve the ethical ideal and exceptions to this general principle may have to be accepted. . . ."[14] The chief exception is stated as follows, under the heading "Social/Cultural Factors":

> In rare circumstances, it may be necessary for researchers to conform to local custom and request partner agreement. An example would be the impossibility of recruiting any research subjects for a study in a particular country without partner agreement and the subsequent impossibility of gaining approval in that country for a new contraceptive drug or device. If failure to conduct the research would result in an inability of people in that country to receive the benefits of the drug or device, this consequence might be judged as sufficiently negative for the common good of the public to outweigh the usual prohibition against partner agreement for the individual subject.[15]

This rationale is often disapprovingly referred to as "the end justifying the means." Yet it is important to note several points about the rationale for this exception. It certainly does not allow an individual to enroll a spouse in research without the spouse's own informed consent to participate. Moreover, the rationale does not endorse the general practice of partner agreement. On the contrary, these guidelines state explicitly that partner agreement "violates the autonomy of research subjects and their right to confidentiality." As a matter of principle, to require partner agreement as a condition of women's participation in research is not ethically acceptable, and these guidelines uphold the principle. The guidelines do not assert that partner agreement should be permitted because in some cultures that is the custom or the norm. Rather, the guidelines justify the exception on grounds that a denial of the eventual benefits of the research to the entire society would be so great as to outweigh the usual prohibition against partner agreement for the individual subject.

This is quite clearly a utilitarian justification. Its use in this context demonstrates the difference between the universality of ethical principles and the very different idea of "absolute" or "exceptionless" principles. The principle of respect for persons is universally applicable, which means that it does not apply only to those countries or cultures whose customs and laws support it. It is not "absolute" in the sense that exceptions cannot ever be countenanced. Special circumstances can justify overriding individual autonomy just as they justify abrogating certain individual rights in other situations. Yet this is a very different ethical justification from one derived from ethical relativism. The relativist justification would be that in cultures where women may not make independent decisions, researchers must adhere to that custom and obtain spousal permission before recruiting women into studies.

Signing Consent Forms: A Procedural Requirement

The requirement in U.S. research regulations that informed consent be documented in a written, signed form points to another example of cross-cultural differences. Especially in social science research, but in some biomedical research as well, researchers in other countries often balk at this requirement. Obtaining written, signed consent forms is sometimes described as an ethical "standard" that is acceptable in the United States but not in other cultures. If researchers in countries where people are reluctant to put their signature on "official" documents use oral consent only, are they adhering to a lower standard, one that is ethically questionable, if not unethical?

A social scientist from a Latin American country told me that the "problem of ethics" is introduced from the outside into her country.[16] When she was studying for her advanced degree in social science, topics in research ethics included the need to preserve anonymity or confidentiality of subjects, the rule that subjects should not be paid (although now social science researchers do pay subjects), and the dictate that social scientists should not make value judgments. What is new are the need to obtain written, informed consent, the requirement to introduce the idea of voluntariness of participation, the idea that subjects can stop the interview at any time, and that they do not have to answer all questions. She emphasized that people in her country do not want to sign anything. This researcher said that the World Health Organization "requires the signed piece of paper" in research that it sponsors. However, she admitted, researchers simply do not adhere to that requirement in their social science studies.

In some situations, strict adherence to the requirement that written consent be obtained would throw up a barrier to carrying out the research. At meetings and in interviews, many researchers in Latin America stated that people in their countries believe they are signing away their rights; or they may view signing a consent form as a "waiver" of some sort. Especially in countries that have until recently had authoritarian or military governments, people are wary of signing papers. According to social scientists I met with in more than one country, written consent is virtually never obtained for social and behavioral studies.

The procedure of obtaining written, signed consent is just that—a procedural requirement and not an ethical "standard." It is not a substitute for the consent process, and there may be ethically sound reasons for waiving this procedural requirement. One obvious reason is that the presence of a signed consent form places the subjects at risk. Social scientists conducting abortion research in the Philippines said that one reason written consent is not obtained is the need to preserve confidentiality. In places where abortion is illegal, the existence of a signed consent form in abortion research reveals the likelihood that the woman had an abortion. The same point was made in Chile by a group carrying out epidemiological research on AIDS. If the very existence of signed consent forms places subjects at risk of psychological, social, or legal harm, then it is not only ethically permissible, but ethically desirable to forego signed consent forms. This is true in the United States as well as in those countries less accustomed to obtaining written consent for participation in research.

Another obvious reason for waiving the requirement for written consent is that some studies involve illiterate subjects. The fact that people are illiterate may not be grounds for disqualifying them, and it is certainly not grounds for abandoning an oral explanation and gaining their permission to serve as subjects. It is, however, sufficient reason to abandon the need for a written document describing what they have been told and requiring that they make an X on a signature line.

The key distinction here is between the process of informing and obtaining voluntary consent from prospective subjects and the piece of paper they are asked to sign. The latter is a consent document, it is not informed consent. It is amazing but true that even today many sophisticated professionals from Western countries continue to fail to distinguish between the process of obtaining people's permission to invade their bodies or ask intrusive questions, on the one hand, and the consent form that is intended to document that process, on the other. They also frequently misconstrue the purpose of an informed consent document. Many physicians believe that the purpose of informed consent is to protect the researcher or clinician from legal liability, and they cynically observe that "you can be sued anyway, so informed consent is not worth the paper it's written on." But this is radically to mistake the purpose. The informed consent document is meant to attest to the research subject's having been told what the researcher plans to do and having granted permission for the research maneuver.

Confidentiality and Privacy

The need to protect the confidentiality of research subjects and respect their privacy is another ethical requirement in Western countries that is often less well established in non-Western cultures. An example from the Philippines illustrates the need to educate social scientists about ethical requirements for research that may depart from other cultural norms of the society in which they live. In a workshop devoted to ethics and social science research, a researcher asked a question about her role in an abortion study. Abortion is illegal in the Philippines and widely thought of as a "sin" in that overwhelmingly Roman Catholic society. The research subject was a widow living with the mother of her deceased husband. The woman had had an abortion after becoming pregnant in an affair. The researcher, about to make a follow-up visit, wondered whether she had an obligation to disclose the woman's abortion to the mother-in-law because it is common practice for everyone in the family to know everyone else's business.

Even if members of the Filipino culture might defend this action outside the research setting, it is surely unacceptable for the researcher to divulge these personal facts. Because the social scientist would not otherwise have access to this information but for the research she was conducting, to disclose information about the research subject's sexual behavior and subsequent illegal abortion to the mother of her deceased husband could potentially harm her interests. It is not only the researcher's obligation to preserve confidentiality that requires nondisclosure, but also the obligation to minimize harm to subjects. This is not a peculiarly "Western" idea or one that can properly be thought of as "ethical imperialism" stemming from U.S. research regulations. The international standards are designed to protect research subjects from harm, whatever local or cultural customs might otherwise permit. When a society's norms and customs diverge from the basic principles of research ethics, researchers are obligated to adhere to the research ethics and not to local or cultural customs.

Two obvious examples illustrate the harm that may befall individuals if family members learn they are participants in research. The first is in HIV research, where even the knowledge that a person is a research subject is likely to reveal the individual's HIV-positive status, a disclosure that could often be harmful to that person's interests. The second example is that of contraceptive research because a woman's mother-in-law or husband could cause trouble for her if they oppose her use of contraceptives. The woman's enrollment in the research study might have been the only way she could gain access to contraceptives. As in the case of HIV research, breach of confidentiality could result in harm. The ethical relativist, adhering to the cultural norm that requires a husband's or a mother-in-law's involvement, would have to accept that prospect of harm to the woman, possibly arguing that greater harm would result from a departure of the cultural tradition of sharing information with the family.

A researcher in Egypt provided two examples of breach of confidentiality for research purposes.[17] In the first case, he was involved in a followup study of family planning services. As part of that study he went to a village where there was a facility operated by the U.S. Agency for International Development. The physician–researcher was not permitted to meet with women in the village, but instead met with the director of the clinic where the women came for family planning services. When the researcher asked the clinic director if women come from surrounding villages to use the services, the director brought out the files of two women from the village. The director did not ask for a letter of authorization from the researcher and without a moment's hesitation gave him the files to peruse for 1 hour. As the researcher described it: "I had access to everything about these women. Anyone could have had access to those women's files."

In telling this story, the Egyptian physician emphasized the fact that the director had not asked him for a letter of authorization or for some other proof of who he was. I asked whether if that had been done would there then have been no ethical problem with the director making the files available? Why should a letter of authorization, showing that the visitor was a researcher, allow him access to personal medical files of women when the researcher was not connected with their medical care? The physician was very thoughtful in making his response and acknowledged that even a letter of authorization, giving him access to the files, would raise an ethical question about breach of confidentiality. It is so common in his country for medical personnel to open their files to researchers that this physician had not considered that having a letter of authorization would not solve the more fundamental ethical problem— that of looking at personal medical files without the permission of the patient.

His second example was one in which research had been conducted on children with learning disabilities. When the research results were published, the article included identifying information about the children. The physician who provided the example criticized the failure to preserve the confidentiality of research subjects in published reports, but in the ensuing discussion participants described this as the norm. They said that medical confidentiality is almost nonexistent in Egypt.

So we return again to the question of ethical relativism. Are the research practices described above—in the Philippines, South America, Egypt, and elsewhere—ones that derive from cultural values in those countries and therefore demand respect? Do they represent adherence to research norms in those countries that represent a cultural difference from what is acceptable in the United States and Western Europe? I think the situation is very much the same as the norms of disclosure and informed consent in the doctor–patient relationship discussed in Chapter 4. The Egyptian physician who described the episodes of breach of confidentiality criticized them and did not attempt to defend them based on "Egyptian ethical principles." The social scientist from the South American country lamented some of the changes she has experienced in research ethics over the years, but she did not rely on "South American ethical principles" in defending the older version of social science ethics. As for the Filipino social scientist who thought it her duty to inform the mother of a woman's deceased husband that the woman had had sex and undergone an abortion, it is worth noting that the other Filipino participants at the workshop were horrified that their colleague would think it appropriate to reveal this piece of confidential information, obtained in the course of research, to the research subject's family.

Relativity of Judgments

What, then, are we entitled to conclude about the statement of universality in research ethics: "If it is unethical to carry out a type of research in one part of the world, it is unethical to do that research in another part of the world"? The statement does appear to mandate uniform ethical standards for research. But to understand just what it permits or rules out requires much interpretation. Especially when the risk-benefit ratios of research studies differ significantly from one part of the world to another, it can lead to controversy. It is not the cultural relativity of values that poses the problem in these cases, but rather the different facts and circumstances on which the ethical judgments rest. Two situations that have sparked considerable controversy illustrate this point. In the first, the quinacrine affair, critics contend that it is ethically unacceptable to use an experimental treatment in developing countries when that same treatment is not approved as safe in developed countries. In their attempted justification, proponents of its use in developing countries point to the difference in risk-benefit ratios.

The Quinacrine Affair

Quinacrine, a drug known to have antimalarial properties, has the effect of producing blockage of the fallopian tubes, and for this reason it is being used as a method of sterilization in some parts of the world.[18] However, quinacrine has not been approved for use as a method for sterilizing women by any national drug regulation authority in the world. Despite the absence of appropriate studies demonstrating that the drug is safe for use in women as a medical method of sterilization, it has been used extensively in Brazil and a number of countries in Asia, including Pakistan, India, Bangladesh, China, Indonesia, and the Philippines. In Vietnam alone, quinacrine has been used to sterilize more than 31,000 women.[19] As of late 1994, an estimated 70,000 women in these and other developing countries have had pellets of quinacrine inserted into their uterus. Appropriate toxicological testing of quinacrine administered in this way is lacking, and scientists do not know exactly how the drug affects the fallopian tube.[20]

Physicians in the United States are permitted by law to use a drug that has been approved for one therapeutic purpose for a different purpose in treating their patients. An underlying presumption, however, is that adequate phase I studies, in which drugs are tested for safety, have been carried out. However, drug manufacturers may not label a drug as indicated for a particular purpose unless the substance has been tested in phase II and phase III studies, which test the drug for its efficacy for particular purposes. If the route of administration of a drug is different from that of the approved use, physicians who prescribe the drug for their patients could be putting those patients at some risk, as well as placing themselves at risk for legal liability. These rules apply in the United States as well as in most developed countries. Some developing countries are largely or entirely lacking in any scheme for regulating the testing, labeling, and use of medications.[21]

The quinacrine affair illustrates one variation in ethical standards as seen from a global perspective. The situation does not involve the actual conduct in developing countries of research that would be considered unacceptable in developed countries. Instead, it is a case of an unapproved drug being introduced into general use before adequate research is completed. While it would be rare for that to happen in the United States, because of both the FDA regulatory system and the physicians' fear of liability, no such barriers or safeguards exist in many developing countries. In effect, the use of quinacrine has become standard therapeutic practice instead of remaining an experimental procedure until adequate testing has been completed.

A number of international organizations addressed this situation. In 1993 the International Planned Parenthood Federation's International Medical Advisory Panel stated that "until the toxicological situation has been clarified and further clinical trials have been conducted, the use of quinacrine pellets for female sterilisation in family planning programs cannot be recommended."[22] A consensus emerged in 1994 from meetings of Family Health International and other organizations that no further clinical trials should take place nor should the drug be prescribed for women until toxicological and retrospective studies have been completed.

Despite all these reservations, quinacrine has continued to have supporters, even among some prestigious members of the world medical community. The British medical journal *Lancet* published an editorial in April 1994 advocating the use of quinacrine in developing countries, where clinicians have continued to provide it. The grounds for advocacy are that the drug is inexpensive and easy to administer, and, especially in situations where few or no other choices exist, it is allegedly safer than undergoing pregnancy. Thus, it is argued, quinacrine is better than nothing for women in those countries. The Scientific and Ethical Review Group of the Special Programme of Research, Development and Research Training in Human Reproduction at the World Health Organization (WHO) issued a statement calling for toxicology testing of quinacrine before any further studies can be carried out in women.[23] In addition, the statement asked that retrospective studies of the women already treated with quinacrine be continued and completed. The director of the WHO program wrote a letter to the *Lancet* saying that "The high standards of safety demanded in the testing and use of contraceptives should apply whether the subjects recruited to the studies are from the developed or the developing world."[24]

In reply to the WHO's insistence on using the same standards for the developed and developing world, one of the leading advocates and users of quinacrine, Dr. Elton Kessel, published a commentary in the *Lancet*. After dismissing the WHO position as "feminist concerns" (presumably, for Kessel, a bad thing), he went on to argue for a double standard on safety and efficacy in the use of risk-benefit ratios. He wrote:

> A simple guide to determining benefits is the estimate for rural areas of South countries that each sterilisation prevents two births. If maternal mortality is, say 3.8 per 1000 live births as estimated for Vietnam, then each 1000 sterilisations done by a new method such as quinacrine pellets will prevent 7.6 maternal deaths. No one has suggested that the method could kill that number of women. . . .[25]

Rebuttals to Kessel's argument take several forms. One rebuttal contends that his position is scientifically flawed because the risks and benefits of a sterilization should be compared only with those of other sterilization methods and not with the risks of pregnancy and childbirth. This is because alternatives to pregnancy exist other than quinacrine sterilization.[26] A different line of rebuttal holds that, according to Kessel's logic, "everyone should be sterilised so that there would be no risk of maternal deaths at all."[27] Most pertinent to ethical relativism is the matter of applying the same or different standards of safety and efficacy to developed and developing countries. One critic of Kessel's view notes that the double standard he defends has been rejected and condemned by the women's health movement, North and South, for many years: "It is precisely the demand for one standard of safety and efficacy for all women that decimates any justification for using quinacrine in women in developing countries, at least at this time."[28]

Given Kessel's dismissal of "feminist concerns" in his reply to the WHO, he is unlikely to care much about gender injustice arising from treating women differently in developed and developing countries. But neither does the defense of quinacrine as an ethically acceptable treatment for women in developing countries rely on cultural factors. The "ethical relativism" in the quinacrine affair takes a different form, one that has nothing to do with cultural diversity. It is a question of whether the assessment of risks and benefits, against a backdrop of poverty and lack of access to medical benefits enjoyed in wealthier countries, can justify lower standards of safety in disadvantaged parts of the world.

Placebo-Controlled HIV/AIDS Clinical Trials

A second controversy also stemmed from different factors that affected the risk-benefit ratio. The debate centered on the ethics of doing a study in a developing country that would be unethical in a developed country. In the quinacrine story, one side argued that different risk-benefit ratios provide ethical warrant for the use of an incompletely researched drug in a developing country, whereas it would not be ethically acceptable to use the unapproved drug in a developed country. The relevant ethical principle is "Treat like cases alike, and different cases differently—in relevant respects."

The key to applying this principle lies in determining what are the relevant respects in which the cases are alike or different. That problem was one of the factors that contributed to a furious controversy that surrounded a set of maternal-to-child transmission studies of HIV carried out in several developing countries in which some research subjects were given placebos. An extended public debate, some of which took place in the pages of the *New England Journal of Medicine*, involved the sponsors of the research—the National Institutes of Health (NIH), the CDC, and the UNAIDS program of AIDS research and their opponents who criticized the studies.[29]

The furor was prompted by an open letter addressed to U.S. officials by the Public Citizen's Health Research Group, which compared the CDC and NIH-sponsored trials to the infamous Tuskegee experiments[30] and newspaper stories that followed. The Public Citizen's advocacy group argued that a proven treatment regimen can reduce the rate of vertical transmission, so it is unethical to withhold that treatment from women in the trial. The proven regimen (known as "076" from the clinical trial in the United States that demonstrated its effectiveness) uses a high dose of AZT, begun midway through pregnancy and administered intravenously to the woman during childbirth. The international collaborative studies were carried out in developing countries that cannot afford the expensive "076" AZT treatment routinely used in the United States and European countries. These clinical trials were testing a lower dose of AZT, which was much cheaper and therefore presumed to be affordable to the poorer countries that would make it available to pregnant women. The developing country studies also began AZT treatment much later in pregnancy because women in those parts of the world do not routinely receive early prenatal care, and the AZT was administered orally rather than intravenously, in line with the availability of medical facilities. These departures from the proven 076 treatment regimen were made in order to adapt AZT for pregnant women to the medical realities in the developed countries where the treatment would be introduced.

For ethical reasons, placebo-controlled trials testing this experimental treatment regimen could not be conducted in the United States. Once its efficacy had been established, the 076 AZT regimen became the standard treatment for HIV-positive pregnant women in the United States and other developed countries. It would surely be unethical to withhold from women in a research study an effective treatment they could obtain as part of their routine medical care. It is evident that these studies did violate the somewhat simple rule: "If it is unethical to carry out a research study in a developed country, it is unethical to do that same research in a developing country." But it is not nearly as clear that these studies violated the formal principle of justice that says: "Treat like cases alike (and different cases differently)." This universal principle of justice lacks content, and, like other abstract universal principles, it requires interpretation for specific applications. The key to applying this principle is determining the relevant respects in which cases are alike or different. Therein lies the dispute over the ethics of the experimental AZT clinical trials in developing countries.

The Public Citizen's group contended that "at least 1002 newborn babies will die as a result of HIV infections they will contract from their mothers in unethical experiments funded by the NIH or the CDC. An additional 502 infants can be expected to die in six other experiments funded by foreign governments including Belgium, Denmark, France, the UN-AIDS program, and South Africa." The group argued that these deaths are unnecessary because women in trials on vertical transmission should be given the treatment regimen proven to reduce the incidence of HIV infection acquired through vertical transmission. Sponsors of the trials replied by noting that more than 350,000 children get infected from perinatal transmission every year in developing countries. It is expected that a shorter regimen would decrease the transmission rate by 40%–50%. Therefore, every year delay in getting the results of these studies implies that 140,000–170,000 children are going to be infected without having access to any intervention.

The reply by the sponsoring agencies to their critics had four parts: (1) the "standard of care" for HIV-positive women in these developing countries is no treatment at all, so they are not being made worse off by being in the study; (2) a placebo-controlled trial can be carried out with many fewer subjects and completed in a much shorter time than can an AZT-controlled study, so useful information pertinent to this population will be available much sooner; (3) the AZT treatment regimen that has become standard in the West is not now and will never be available to this population because of its prohibitive costs, so its use in a research study cannot be justified; (4) if it is proven to be effective, the much cheaper and more appropriate experimental regimen will be made available by governments to all pregnant women in these countries. The conclusion defenders of these trials reached is that thousands more children's lives will be saved by conducting the shorter, placebo-controlled trial than by the longer, AZT-controlled study,[31] so it is ethical to do the placebo-controlled study in those countries.

Public Citizen's Health Research Group sought to rebut the argument, claiming that the research violates at least 4 of the 10 principles of the Nuremberg Code, and, in addition, Guideline 15 of the International Ethical Guidelines for Biomedical Research involving Human Subjects[32] is violated. That Guideline states that the ethical standards of the sponsoring agency's country should prevail when research is conducted in another country and that the ethical standards should be no less exacting than those in the sponsoring agency's country.[33] The Public Citizen's group claimed that because these trials could not be conducted in developed countries today, the researchers "have chosen to ignore these standards of ethical conduct accepted the world over and have sunk to standards below those acceptable in their home countries." A different, and lower standard was being applied to poor, developing countries than that employed in wealthier countries, and, they argued, that constituted an unacceptable ethical relativism.

The opponents in this dispute could both claim that justice was on their side. The Public Citizen's group began with the premise that the same study could not ethically be carried out in developed countries and concluded that, therefore, it would be unethical to conduct it in developing countries. The sponsoring agencies began with the premise that risk-benefit ratios are radically different in developing countries and in the sponsoring agencies' countries. In the developed countries, all women potentially had access to the effective treatment regimen but in the developing countries none did. In the developing countries, subjects were not being placed at greater risk than if they were not in the study at all, and many more people could potentially benefit much sooner from the shorter, placebo-controlled trial. The two cases were therefore not similar, but different in relevant respects, so the principle of justice—"treat like cases alike"—was not violated.

Defenders of the placebo-controlled trials included representatives from the developing countries in which the trials were conducted. Some argued that the studies were ethically acceptable because they satisfied the relevant procedural requirements for approving and conducting research. They pointed out that the placebo-controlled perinatal transmission studies were approved by ethical review committees in the developed countries that sponsored the trials and also in the developing countries where they were being conducted. Furthermore, they argued, researchers from the developing countries were carrying out the studies in their own countries, and women enrolled in the studies granted their voluntary, informed consent to participate. Therefore, they concluded, because the placebo-controlled trials adhered to ethically adequate procedures, they are ethically acceptable. Based on the approval of health officials in his country, as well as local ethical review and approval, one African researcher remarked that the Public Citizen's critique of these AIDS trials "reeks of ethical imperialism."

This controversy has all the earmarks of a genuine ethical dilemma. The research in question does appear to violate a condition stated in the international Declaration of Helsinki: "In any medical study, every patient—including those of a control group, if any—should be assured of the best proven diagnostic and therapeutic method."[34] In the placebocontrolled studies, no group is provided with the best proven therapeutic method. However, Robert J. Levine, an expert in the ethics of human subjects research, questioned the interpretation of the phrase "the best proven treatment": "When Helsinki calls for the 'best proven therapeutic method' does it mean the 'best therapy available anywhere in the world'? Or does it mean the standard that prevails in the country in which the trial is conducted?" Levine's answer is that "the best proven therapy standard must necessarily mean the standard that prevails in the country in which the clinical trial is carried out."[35]

Others argue that to adopt that standard is to exploit nations and people who are economically disadvantaged. One physician writes: "Exploitation by industrialized countries of the human and natural resources of the developing world has a long and tragic history. It has never been difficult for economically wealthy countries to justify their acts by citing, for example, the supposed genetic or moral inferiority of those exploited. Substituting economic inferiority in these old arguments makes the enterprise no less offensive."[36]

The placebo arm of these studies was suspended in Thailand and Ivory Coast in February 1998, when results demonstrated the unquestioned superiority of the short course of AZT over placebo. But the early completion of the trials did not end the debate between medical scientists and ethicists who had staked out positions on either side. It would be a mistake, however, to view this ethical controversy as one that involved a tension between cultural relativism and ethical universalism. The controversy had little to do with different norms or values in different countries and everything to do with the economic disparity between developed and developing countries. Resulting from that economic disparity is a different standard of medical care in wealthier countries and poorer nations. As one observer noted, "the real double standard lies not in the way the trials are being conducted, but in the inequity in access to medicines in different countries."[37]

What the defenders of the placebo-controlled trials took to be relative was the risk-benefit ratio of the study. The trials had a different risk-benefit ratio in Thailand, Ivory Coast, and Uganda than the same research design would have had in the United States. What the critics of the trials took to be nonrelative were the ethical principles stated in several international guidelines. Although combatants in this controversy hurled charges and countercharges of "ethical exploitation" and "ethical imperialism," the debate had nothing to do with whether ethical standards should be relativized to culture.

A question of procedural ethics remained unresolved in this episode of international collaborative research. The Ugandan researcher who claimed that the stance of the Public Citizen's group "reeked of ethical imperialism" argued that researchers from Uganda and representatives from the Ugandan Ministry of Health were full participants in the decision to initiate the trials. This view maintains that people from a given culture or country are in the best position to decide what is best for their country, not some outsiders who are unrelated to the research and unfamiliar with the health needs of the region. Furthermore, local ethical committees reviewed and approved the research. Because these trials were preceded by proper procedures, involving local and regional committees and officials, they must therefore be ethically acceptable.

However, adherence to proper procedures is not sufficient to guarantee substantive ethical results. A properly constituted ethical review committee might still approve a piece of ethically unsound research. One reply to the procedural justification addressed its weakness: "Since the Tuskegee study was conducted by Americans on Americans, this argument obviously does not stand. . . . Unethical research will not benefit developing countries in the long run, since it undermines human rights, which are the very foundation on which sustainable development needs to be built."[38]

Does unethical research, by virtue of its being unethical, violate human rights? If research is unethical, either it violates an ethical principle governing research or it fails to comply with proper procedures mandated for conducting research. Whether a research study or a type of medical practice is unethical is one question. It must be kept distinct from the question whether unethical research or medical practice violates *human rights*. That question takes us into the important but murky area of defining and circumscribing the realm of human rights.

Notes

1. Emily Miller, "International Trends in Ethical Review of Medical Research," *IRB: A Review of Human Subjects Research*, Vol. 3 (October 1981), p. 9.

2. Miller, p. 10.

3. Sue V. Rosser, "Research Bias," (ed.) Warren T. Reich, *Encyclopedia of Bioethics*, 2nd edition (New York: Macmillan Library Reference, 1995), pp. 2261–2266.

4. See also P. Vaughan, *The Pill on Trial* (New York: Coward and Macann, 1970).

5. Donald Warwick, "Contraceptives in the Third World," *Hastings Center Report* Vol. 5 (1975), p. 9.

6. Warwick, p. 9.

7. The researcher was present at a conference devoted to ethics and research held at the University Of North Carolina, Chapel Hill, North Carolina, in November 1995.

8. Lisa H. Newton, "Ethical Imperialism and Informed Consent," *IRB: A Review of Human Subjects Research*, Vol. 12 (May/June 1990), p. 11.

9. Carel B. Ijsselmuiden and Ruth R. Faden, "Images in Clinical Medicine," *New England Journal of Medicine*, Vol. 326 (1992), p. 833.

10. These details and the correspondence were provided to me by the program officer in connection with my role as a temporary adviser to the program. Names and insititutions are omitted here to protect confidentiality.

11. This episode was related to me during my visit to Bangladesh as part of my Ford Foundation Project in March 1994.

12. Sana Loue, David Okello, Medi Kawuma, "Research Bioethics in the Ugandan Context: A Program Summary," *Journal of Law, Medicine & Ethics*, Vol. 24, No. 1 (1996), pp. 47–53.

13. Scientific and Ethical Review Group, Special Programme of Research, Development, and Research Training in Human Reproduction, World Health Or-

ganization, *Guidelines on Reproductive Health Research and Partners' Agreement* (unpublished), p. 3.

14. Scientific and Ethical Review Group, p. 2.

15. Scientific and Ethical Review Group, p. 2.

16. This was recounted during my visit to South America, in September-October 1995, as part of my Ford Foundation Project.

17. This was recounted during my visit to Egypt in January 1996, as part of my Ford Foundation project.

18. UNDP/UNFPA/WHO/World Bank Special Programme of Research, Development and Research Training in Human Reproduction, *Progress in Human Reproduction Research*, 31 (1994), p. 4; Marge Berer, "The Quinacrine Controversy One Year On," *Reproductive Health Matters*, No. 4 (November 1994), pp. 99–106.

19. Berer, pp. 103–104.

20. UNDP/UNFPA/WHO/World Bank Special Programme.

21. One such country is Brazil. During a visit I made to that country in April 1996, several people told me that "control of medications is chaotic in Brazil" (Ford Foundation project on Ethics and Reproductive Health).

22. Berer, p. 99.

23. Scientific review body voices concern at use of quinacrine for sterilization," *Progress in Human Reproduction Research*, Vol. 31 (1994), p. 8.

24. Giuseppe Benagiano, "Sterilisation by Quinacrine" (Letter)," *Lancet*, Vol. 344 (September 3, 1994), p. 689.

25. Elton Kessel, "Quinacrine Sterilisation Revisited" (Commentary), *Lancet*, Vol. 344 (1994), pp. 698–700.

26. Berer, p. 100.

27. Berer, p. 100.

28. Berer, p. 100.

29. In addition to the sources cited, some of the positions and arguments desribed in this section are taken from discussions, meetings, and conferences in which I participated while the debate was going on.

30. Public Citizen News Release, Media Advisory, April 22, 1997.

31. David Brown, "Medical Group Condemns US AIDS Drug Tests in Africa for Using Placebo," *Washington Post* (April 23, 1997).

32. Public Citizen, open letter to Secretary Donna Shalala, April 22, 1997, pp. 3, 10.

33. Council for International Organizations of Medical Sciences (CIOMS) in collaboration with the World Health Organization (WHO), *International Ethical Guidelines for Biomedical Research Involving Human Subjects* (Geneva, 1993), p. 43.

34 Declaration of Helsinki, Article II. 3.

35. Robert J. Levine, "The 'Best Proven Therapeutic Method' Standard in Clinical Trials in Technologically Developing Countries," *IRB: A Review of Human Subjects Research*, Vol. 20, No. 1 (1998), p. 6.

36. Roy J. Kim, "Letter to the Editor," *New England Journal of Medicine*, Vol. 338, No. 12 (1998), p. 838.

37. Peter Piot, "Letter to the Editor," *New England Journal of Medicine*, Vol. 228, No. 12 (1998), p. 839.

38. Carel B. IJsselmuiden, "Letter to the Editor," *New England Journal of Medicine*, Vol. 228, No. 12 (1998), p. 838.

9

Human Rights

in

Health

and

Medicine

I T is indisputable that the experiments conducted by German doctors during the Nazi era were gross violations of the human rights of their victims. If anything counts as a *human* right—one that is universally applicable to all humans—it is the right not to be forced to undergo medical experiments intended to result in death. However, the sweeping claim that unethical research undermines human rights signals a move from charging that something is unethical to alleging that it is a violation of a moral standard of the highest order. Although it is true that research subjects have rights that deserve protection, an additional argument is needed to show that the rights of research subjects should be classified under the heading of "human" rights.

In an article entitled "Human Experimentation and Human Rights," Jay Katz acknowledges that the contours of human rights are still ill-defined.[1] Yet Katz cites the many United Nations resolutions on human rights in support of his contention that current research regulations in the United States fail to protect the *human* rights of subjects of research. He asserts that research subjects possess human rights that are inviolate, but stops short of providing a full-blown argument linking the concept of human rights with the rights of research subjects. The closest he comes is to invoke the idea that "human beings possess rights to inviolate dignity."[2] However, appeals to human dignity are not intuitively more clear than appeals to human rights. If anything, they are more obscure.

European pronouncements on ethics and medicine often make the concept of human dignity the centerpiece of declarations and conventions involving rights. To take one example, the Council of Europe issued a Convention on Human Rights and Biomedicine entitled "Convention for the Protection of Human rights and Dignity of the Human Being with Regard to the Application of Biology and Medicine."[3] The convention emphasizes "the importance of ensuring the dignity of the human being" and observes that "the misuse of biology and medicine may lead to acts endangering human dignity."[4] Nowhere does the document explain what is meant in this context by "human dignity."

Other appeals to human dignity followed in the wake of the announcement early in 1997 that Scottish scientists had succeeded in cloning the first mammal, Dolly the sheep. A British commentator observed that the reports from France and Germany, which were issued very quickly after the cloning news broke, suffered from dogmatism and overused the rhetoric of cloning being "an attack on human dignity."[5] Although the concept of human dignity can have a legitimate place in ethical discourse in connection with cloning, genetic manipulations, and other biomedical activities, more precision is required than simply asserting that "human dignity is violated." If human dignity is a vague concept, its basis for claims about human rights is even more obscure.

As recounted in Chapter 7, a movement to treat reproductive rights as a species of human rights gained momentum in the period surrounding the United Nations conferences in Cairo and Beijing. More generally, scholars and women's health advocates have sought the promotion and protection of women's health through international human rights law.[6] Others have connected human rights with the AIDS pandemic, arguing that the protection of human rights is necessary to decrease vulnerability to HIV infection and to eliminate all forms of discrimination against people living with HIV/AIDS.[7] A new journal devoted to health and human rights was founded in 1994, and in still another development the International Bioethics Committee of UNESCO drafted a "universal declaration on the human genome and human rights" in 1997.

When a moral claim is cast in terms of human rights, it commands the attention of governments and citizens throughout the world. It also compels the need for a response on the part of those accused of violating human rights. Governments, military personnel, antigovernment rebels, and other groups accused of violating human rights typically react with one of two very different responses. Either they acknowledge the existence and importance of human rights and deny that their own actions are, in fact, violations of those rights; or they reject altogether the concept of rights as a Western idea that does not apply to their culture or region of the world. The latter response is a classic reliance on ethical relativism. It cuts off further debate on the details of the alleged violation by asserting that the category of rights (and, with it, the subcategory of human rights) is inapplicable to their country or region.

The former response—admission of the category of human rights but denial that the action in question is, indeed, a violation—requires a probing analysis of human rights. Should the concept of human rights be limited to items found in declarations and conventions that are among the elements of international human rights law? Is the concept of human rights properly applied only to a subcategory of moral rights—those deemed to have the highest importance? Is the significance attached to human rights diminished when the concept is broadened indiscriminately? To undertake such a comprehensive analysis would be a major project, well beyond the scope of what can be accomplished here. I will focus instead on the more modest task of exploring appeals to human rights made in a variety of medical and health care contexts. Inevitably, this task will involve references to the larger scope of human rights, their articulation in various international conventions and declarations, as well as in ordinary discourse.

The Language of Rights

It is commonplace for Westerners to use the language of rights to make all sorts of general claims that pertain to obligations of government, to relations among people, and between individuals and institutions such as schools, businesses, and hospitals. But rights language is still far from universal as ethical currency. A women's health activist in the Philippines said there is no idea of reproductive rights among the rural women she works with and not even a concept of women's rights more generally.[8] Attempts by women's health advocates to frame ethical concerns relating to women's health in the language of rights have not been successful in that setting, despite the embodiment of rights in constitutional and civil law in the Philippines. Two women's health advocates in Brazil made a similar point. They said that in the poor region outside the city of Recife, where their clinic is located, people do not have any rights and do not think in terms of rights. They are worried about survival. In these and other parts of the world, rights are simply not part of the moral vocabulary.

Yet even in countries where advocates of human rights have a strong voice because of past abuses by military regimes and authoritarian governments, some people criticize what they take to be the overuse of rights language in the United States. A social science researcher from Argentina, re-marking on what she perceived to be the extremes accorded to the status of the individual in the United States, expressed the view that Americans are "so worried about individual rights." But, she mused, other things are more important. I found this rather surprising, especially because Argentina has lived through many years of military rule and political oppression, ending only in the 1980s with a democratically elected government. Moreover, this researcher herself is engaged in studies on behalf of an organization that promotes the reproductive rights of women.

A Chinese scholar made a similar point about rights talk: "In the West rights talks seem to be extended to everything: patient's right, fetus' right, embryo's right, fertilized egg's right, seriously defective newborn's right, very low birthweight infant's right, irreversibly comatose's right, patient in persistent vegetative state's right, dead body's right, and animal right, vegetation's right, and so on."[9] Interestingly, however, this Chinese professor favors an approach that emphasizes rights, especially in his own country, because of the longstanding cultural tradition that has empha-sized duties without corresponding rights.

When I pressed the Argentine social scientist to say just which indi-vidual rights she thought were overemphasized in the United States, or which ones should be overridden by other values, she was unable to come up with examples. Our conversation was typical of what happens when ex-pressions of libertarian, economic self-interest are confused with the civil and political rights of individuals. It may well be true that reverence for the individual in the United States goes to greater extremes than in other countries, but this does not necessarily translate into an obsessive concern for the rights of individuals.

After considerable discussion and elaboration, it turned out that what the Argentine social scientist really meant was that there is much "rights talk" and many rights claims people make in their day-to-day lives. When confronted directly, as in this conversation, most critics from outside the United States do not deny the paramount importance of the right of indi-viduals not to have the government abridge their liberty, invade their pri-vacy, breach their confidentiality, or deny them freedom of speech and re-ligion. Yet the question remains: Are all these rights properly termed *human* rights, ones that transcend cultural differences and national boundaries, and ought therefore to be respected universally?

A somewhat curious twist is the turning away from the centrality of rights in some contemporary American academic circles, notably among those who call themselves "communitarians" and some feminist theorists. Communitarians avoid rights language because they believe it places too much emphasis on the individual at the expense of the common interests people have in being members of the larger community. It seems odd to find rights language being rejected by authoritarian, patriarchal regimes, such as China or the Vatican, and also by their sometime opponents among feminist thinkers and communitarians in the ivory tower. Feminists surely do not embrace the patriarchy evinced by some leaders of traditional religious communities and by the Pope. And communitarians do not defend the oppression of political dissidents by the authoritarian government in China or military regimes in countries that continue to be ruled by strongmen.

The abuses that have occurred and are still occurring in many parts of the world can be recognized as such and ultimately rectified only by acknowledging the rights of human subjects of research, of patients who undergo unnecessary procedures or suffer complications in the hands of poorly trained physicians, of women in developing countries who are in desperate need of safe and effective methods to control fertility, to mention only a few areas in the biomedical arena in which recognition and protection of individual rights has constituted moral progress.

Critics of the use of rights language argue that an emphasis on self-interest leaves little room for trust, generosity, and community responsibility in matters of health and illness.[10] Yet a glimpse at the use of authority and abuse of power by physicians in many developing countries shows that precisely what is missing is trust, generosity, and community responsibility. No trust is warranted in doctors who do unnecessary procedures in order to earn more money[11] or in governmental authorities that fail to ensure that practicing physicians are competent and appropriately trained.[12] No generosity is evident among doctors who refuse to perform abortions on their patients whom they visit in public hospitals in the morning, while they regularly do the procedure for the paying patients they see in their private offices in the afternoon.[13] In India and Bangladesh, for example, physicians are accountable to no one and engage in malpractice with impunity. Ethically concerned doctors, social workers, and other health practitioners described a system in which medical records and documentation are nonexistent or chaotic, leaving no paper trail for victims of malpractice who have the wherewithal to try to bring a malpractice suit. Even if a patient or family knows enough or has sufficient resources to initiate the process, the attempt soon gets bogged down in the judicial bureaucracy and rarely succeeds in reaching an outcome. Perhaps if American ethicists, feminists, and communitarians who have been critical of the "overuse" of rights language were more aware of the way doctors in countries that lack a tradition of individual rights treat their patients, these critics might become persuaded of the value of using rights language for initiating and sustaining much-needed reforms.

Interpretations of "Human Rights"

The original significance attached to human rights was that they are rights possessed by all individuals everywhere against the state. The concept of human rights was designed to protect individuals from oppressive power and authority wielded by governments, to protect citizens from state actions carried out without due process of law. The following characterization of human rights attempts to capture the central idea.

"*The moral rights of all people in all situations*—This is where human rights fit into the scheme. A human right is something that everybody has. They are not rights a man acquires by doing certain work, enacting a certain role, or discharging certain duties; they belong to him simply because he is a human being."[14] Although this characterization stresses the universality of human rights and takes it beyond the relationship between governments and their citizens, it is framed in language that today would be considered politically incorrect because it refers to *man* rather than to *person*. The irony of this choice of words is that the author of the passage, recounting the history of the concept of human rights, began as follows:

"'Human Rights' is a fairly new name for what were formerly called

'the rights of man.' It was Eleanor Roosevelt in the 1940s who promoted the
use of the expression human rights when she discovered, through her work
in the United Nations, that the rights of men were not understood in some
parts of the world to include the rights of women. The rights of man at an
earlier date had itself replaced the original term 'natural rights.' . . ."[15]

Skepticism about the concept of human rights and its universal application typically resorts to the facts of cultural diversity. An anthropologist
asks: "Are there universal human rights that can be applied without cultural imposition? How is it to be determined what constitutes a violation of
these rights?"[16] In support of her contention that these are difficult questions to answer, the anthropologist cites a "Statement on Human Rights"
published in 1947 in a scholarly journal in her field: "what is held to be a
human right in one society may be regarded as anti-social by another people, or by the same people in a different period of their history."[17] Going
well beyond skepticism to a denial of the very possibility of identifying a
class of human rights is the following statement by two anthropologists referring to the United Nations Charter (1945) and the Universal Declaration of Human Rights (1948):

> '[T]he Western political philosophy upon which the Charter and the
> Declaration are based provides only one particular interpretation of human
> rights, and . . . this Western notion may not be successfully applicable to
> non-Western areas for several reasons: . . . cultural differences whereby
> the philosophic underpinnings defining human nature and the relationship
> of individuals to others and to society are markedly at variance with Western
> individualism.'[18]

These anthropologists conclude that a rethinking of the conception
of human rights is needed.

Thus, in response to the most general question "Are there any human
rights?" anthropologists have expressed three distinct views: "certainly,
yes"; "possibly, but they are hard to identify"; and "not really." These views
about the validity of the concept of human rights exactly mirror the main
positions regarding ethical relativism. The first insists on the legitimacy of
certain fundamental ethical principles, which are held to be universally
valid even if not universally acknowledged. The second can be considered

a form of "ethical pluralism." And the third is the classic version of ethical relativism: Because different cultures do, in fact, subscribe to different ethical norms, these are the only ethical values that can be considered valid for them.

In contrast to the rejection of the universality of human rights by these scholars in anthropology, representatives of nations throughout the world came together and agreed upon the Declaration of Human Rights in 1948. Yet in the more than 50 years that have elapsed since then, debate has persisted over whether both "negative" rights (e.g., the right to be free *from* oppression, *from* governmental interference with liberty of speech and action) and "positive" rights (rights *to* basic goods and services needed to sustain life and health) ought properly to be construed as human rights. Leading illustrations of each type are, first, Article 3, "Everyone has the right to life, liberty, and the security of person" and Article 5, "No one shall be subjected to torture or to cruel, inhuman or degrading treatment or punishment"; and, second, Article 15, "Everyone has the right to a standard of living adequate for the health and well-being of himself," and "Motherhood and childhood are entitled to special care and assistance."[19]

The first category, negative rights, has come under attack from countries that reject this type of right as too "individualistic" and therefore not applicable to their more "communitarian" societies. This objection is voiced by defenders of "Asian values." The second category, "positive rights," has been rejected by American devotees of the capitalist system who oppose the role of government exemplified in the welfare state. Positive rights have also been criticized on the grounds that such rights are impossible to fulfill and are, therefore, statements of ideals rather than rights. In the words of one critic:

> I wish to suggest that one can justify the existence of . . . universal human rights, provided one does not do what the UN did in 1948, and which fashionable opinion has continued to do: that is, to postulate as human rights universal claims to amenities like social security and holidays with pay. Such things are admirable as ideals, but an ideal belongs to a wholly different logical category from a right. If rights are to be reduced to the status of ideals, the whole enterprise of protecting human rights will be sabotaged.[20]

An American philosopher, Maurice Cranston, issued this last objection, so it might be dismissed as arising out of ethnocentric bias in the same way the Asian "communitarian" view rejects values associated with Western individualism. But that would be to ignore the perceptive point of distinguishing between a right that governments can realistically fulfill and a noble ideal that is worth striving for but cannot be fulfilled with the same ease as negative rights. As Cranston points out: "The effect of a universal declaration that is overloaded with affirmations of economic and social rights is to push the political and civil rights out of the realm of the morally compelling into the twilight world of utopian aspirations. . . . [N]othing is more important to an understanding of a right than to acknowledge that a right is *not* an ideal."[21] This argument, as compelling as it is, points to the grave difficulty of defending the claim that health is a human right—a claim we will examine shortly. First, let us take a closer look at the view that "Asian values" are incompatible with human rights.

"Asian Values" and Human Rights

Spokespersons from some developing countries have complained at UN-sponsored world conferences that the concept of rights is a Western or European or North American idea quite alien in other places, especially in Asia and Africa. What we in North America and Europe take for granted ethically, politically, and legally often are not only questioned, but are rejected outright by spokespersons from other cultures. At the United Nations World Conference on Human Rights in 1993 in Vienna, several countries challenged the universality of human rights, maintaining that human rights should be interpreted differently in regions with non-Western cultures. Among the leaders of this challenge were China, Syria, and Iran; others included Singapore, Malaysia, Indonesia, Yemen, Vietnam, and Cuba. Representatives from China, other Asian nations, and Iraq used cultural relativism to defend their governmental actions that Western nations called abuses of human rights. This defense relied on distinguishing between European and American norms, which prohibit the suppression of political dissenters, and the cultural tradition of the East, which stems from Confucian morality.

The argument was made that the ancient cultures of the East have the right to follow their own customs. As one commentator notes: "In some versions of this defense by the Chinese and Singaporean governments, the modern police state becomes an expression of traditional Confucian morality. . . . [T]his whole line of argument . . . grossly libels the very cultures it ostensibly defends by implying that individual rights have no place in them."[22] The then U.S. Secretary of State Warren Christopher, speaking on the opening day of the conference, said: "We cannot let cultural relativism become the last refuge of repression."[23] Pointing to cultural or religious traditions provides, at best, an explanation for suppressing political dissidents by relying on the premise: "Things were always like this in our cultural tradition, so this is why they should continue to be like this." It could only serve as a *justification* if we add the leading premise of normative ethical relativism: "Whatever a culture or tradition deems to be right is, therefore, right for it."

In a later episode, Secretary of State Madeleine Albright clashed with leaders of Malaysia over the 1948 Universal Declaration of Human Rights. The Malaysian Prime Minister said that the declaration had been "formulated by the superpowers, which did not understand the needs of poor countries." He called the West's insistence that developing countries conform to high ideals on human rights "oppressing." Ms. Albright replied that "it would be a great mistake to consider these principles imposed by the West."[24] What Ms. Albright might better have said is that despite the Western origin of the idea of human rights, the concept is one that should apply to all nations, in all parts of the world.

Chinese officials have been among the leading opponents of the universality of human rights, having many times been accused of human rights violations by Western nations. As one scholar explains: "In the field of human rights traditional Chinese political culture and contemporary communist ideology reinforce each other in the denial of political and civil rights, while they converge to promote the satisfaction of the basic needs of the people. They both emphasize the collective instead of the individual and duties instead of rights. . . ."[25]

A more nuanced view of Chinese history confirms the dominant view that places emphasis on satisfaction of the needs of the people and ignores their civil and political rights, but at the same time argues that concern for human rights is neither alien to China nor merely a Western import: "[A]lthough China does not have a tradition of individual liberties and legal rights, it does have one of humane concern, which found its expression in the Confucian literati's criticism of the government for unfair treatment of the population and the abuse of power. Without directly challenging the authoritarian nature of the Confucian system, individuals and groups throughout Chinese history have criticized political oppression and sought to curb despotic rulers, often risking death to protest against government misdeeds and to propose reforms."[26]

Both of the views just cited exemplify the descriptive thesis of cultural relativism, in this case applied to human rights. The descriptive thesis has never been in doubt. The hard question is, what are the implications of the descriptive thesis for the position that human rights cannot be universally applied because the concept of human rights—at least as interpreted and endorsed by Western nations—is inapplicable to nations and cultures in other parts of the world?

That hard question is tackled by still another Chinese scholar, who takes aim at the defense of Asian cultural exceptionalism. Xiaorong Li criticizes the notion that there exists a single, coherent "Asian view" of human rights.[27] He identifies and argues against three leading claims made by spokespersons for Asian governments: Claim I, that rights are "culturally specific"; claim II, that the community takes precedence over individuals; and claim III, that social and economic rights take precedence over individual rights.

In arguing against the first of these claims, Li observes that, in practice, advocates of the "Asian view" fail to adhere to the rule that social norms originating in other cultures should not be adopted in Asian cultures. In fact, Asian leaders freely pick and choose what they like from other cultures, embracing what is in their political interest, such as capitalist economics and consumerist culture.[28] Li argues further that the idea that Asians value community over individuality obscures certain underlying realities by collapsing "community" into the state and the state into the (current) regime.[29] This maneuver makes possible a dismissal of human rights that, if exercised, would come into conflict with the rulers' interests. Li distinguishes between what a true "Confucian communitarian" would favor in the name of social harmony and the oppressive power Chinese leaders wield over dissenters. The latter has little in common with the Confucian idea of social harmony.

Against the third claim of "Asian values"—that economic development rights take precedence over political and civil rights—Li maintains it poses a false dilemma. People need not have to choose between the two miserable options of starvation and oppression. In sum, Li contends, we should not fall prey to the threat posed by "Asian values" to the universality of human rights because the arguments in favor of that perspective are flawed and self-serving tools of leaders seeking to maintain their power by preserving the status quo.

In what may seem like an ironic twist, Chinese officials, responding to an annual report issued by the U.S. State Department on the status of human rights in China, turned the tables and came out with a list of human rights violations in the United States. Included on the list of violations were racism, inequality of the sexes, and money-dominated politics. The Chinese report criticized the U.S. government for turning a blind eye to human rights problems in its own country.[30] This response by Chinese officials is inconsistent with China's repeated insistence that human rights is a Western concept, inapplicable outside those Western countries in which it originated. It would seem that the Chinese cannot have it both ways—denying the legitimacy of the concept and at the same time criticizing the United States for human rights violations. It is evident, however, that an allegation of violations of human rights is a powerful political tool, whoever may choose to wield it.

An obvious way out of this apparent inconsistency is to acknowledge that the concept of human rights is legitimate but to recognize disagreements about which items properly belong on the list of human rights. This is the crux of the debate between Western nations and those that defend "Asian values." Western countries have placed individual freedom at the top of the list, whereas China and other non-Western nations insist that the common good transcends individual rights. The Chinese critique mentioned the very limited human rights protection provided by the U.S. Constitution, noting the absence of a right to "food, clothing, shelter, education, the right to work, rest and reasonable payment."[31] The Chinese might also have noted the absence of a right to health care, a situation that many Westerners, including Americans, take to be an egregious moral omission by the government of the richest nation in the world.

The key difference, then, between the United States and China is their recognition of a different class of rights as human rights. The United States considers human rights to be a subset of the class of "negative" rights: the right of individuals not to be interfered with by the state. In contrast, China largely excludes negative rights (freedom, privacy) and focuses instead on "positive" rights—those that establish an obligation on the part of the government to provide something to its citizens. As noted earlier, the debate over whether positive rights (sometimes called *entitlements* in the United States) ought to be considered human rights has persisted since the enunciation of the Universal Declaration of Human Rights in 1948.

The international discussion of human rights according to "Asian" or "Western" values takes place mainly against the backdrop of two international covenants: the International Covenant on Social, Economic, and Cultural Rights (ICSECR), which the United States has only just signed and has yet to ratify; and the International Covenant on Civil and Political Rights (ICCPR), which China signed in October 1998. Both of these human rights covenants were adopted in 1966, nearly two decades after the UN Declaration of Human Rights. Xiaorong Li observes that although China's continued emphasis on social–economic rights has been endorsed by other Southeast Asian leaders, not all Asians agree.[32] Asian human rights groups have insisted that people must not be forced to give up their civil and political liberty in exchange for a promise of economic well–being. These human rights advocates have been pushing for a "holistic and integrated approach to human rights."[33] Nevertheless, as Li notes, this approach constitutes a departure from the mainstream position of international human rights organizations, which have always assigned priority to civil–political rather than social–economic rights.

Li argues persuasively that the distinction between these two classes of rights cannot be made by viewing the former set of rights as ones that can be immediately implemented and the latter set as ones that can only be progressively realized. Nor can the former be seen as stemming from "absolute" obligations of governments and the latter as arising out of "imperfect" obligations. The two classes of rights also cannot be distinguished according to whether the rights in question would be costly or inexpensive to implement. Rather, it is important to make priority rankings within each of the two sets of human rights and for human rights groups to make a realistic assessment of how they can be most effective in promoting rights in both categories. As Li points out, human rights groups have never contended that the right to free legal counsel (a civil and political right found in the ICCPR) is more important than the right not to starve (a social and economic right stated in the ICSECR).[34] It is hard to think of a right as basic to human health as "the right not to starve."

Human Rights in Medicine and Health

The expansion of the ordinary language of rights to that of human rights has become increasingly widespread in the domain of health and medicine. This expansionist phenomenon is evident among academics who work in the fields of medicine, public health, and bioethics, as well as among health advocates in areas related to AIDS and reproductive health, and beyond. This raises the question of whether all rights related to medicine and health may be classed as human rights or whether the designation "human rights" should be reserved for a specific subset of rights that deserves universal recognition. In one sense the classification of all rights pertaining to human beings is trivially true. If we want to distinguish between rights that apply to members of the species *Homo sapiens* rather than to members of the animal kingdom, all of the former are human rights by definition. But this tautological sense is not what people mean when they argue that the right to health care or the right to health itself is a human right, the right not to be sterilized by the government is a human right, and the right not to have one's genitals cut is a human right.

Both negative and positive rights have been claimed within the domain of medicine and health. The alleged "right to health" is an unabashed positive right, which makes claims on governments to act in a wide variety of ways on behalf of the health of their people. The idea of "reproductive rights" includes a subset of both negative and positive rights.

Consider the following two examples of the somewhat casual replacement of the simple term *rights*, which need not have implications for universality, with the idea of *human rights*, which typically does imply universal applicability. In the first example, a newspaper article discussing insurance coverage for infertility treatments quotes the noted health economist, Uwe E. Reinhardt: "Is having your own offspring with your own genes a matter of human right? And if you can't accomplish that on your own, do you have the right to have your efforts to achieve it financed?"[35] Clearly, if having one's own offspring with one's own genes *is* a human right, and if Mother Nature failed to fulfill that right, individuals do have a claim against insurers or the government lest a human right be violated. The debates in the United States over just which health care services governmental and private insurers should reimburse reflects this nation's ambivalence about positive rights.

In the second example, responding to an article describing a campaign in Peru to sterilize women, a letter to the editor observed that Peru's sterilization campaign was inconsistent with a Peruvian governmental program "which clearly stated that respect for women's human rights should guide reproductive and family planning activities."[36] When a governmental program attempts to impose a measure that renders women permanently incapable of having more children, it is a clear violation of the negative right to remain free from interference with an individual's desire to regulate fertility. That freedom is a more likely candidate for a human right, as it is embodied in international declarations and covenants (see below) despite actions by governments that have continued to maintain strict population control policies.

Health as a Human Right

A deliberate expansion of rights language into the sphere of health was the creation in 1994 of a new international journal, *Health and Human*

Rights. The inaugural issue noted that workers in the disciplines of human rights and health "have begun to see that their goals are complementary; that they face common obstacles; that human rights violations translate directly into morbidity and mortality at the individual and group level. . . ."[37] Although the truth of these empirical observations cannot be denied, and the laudable goal of improving both health and health care throughout the world should have no opponents, a fundamental premise of the journal raises a profound philosophical question. That is whether "the right to health" is a useful practical idea, given at least one leading definition of health and the circumstances that lie beyond human control in contributing to good or bad health.

The leading definition of *health*, often criticized as being overly broad, is from the WHO: "A complete state of physical, mental, and social well-being, and not merely the absence of disease." One criticism is that it defines an ideal that is impossible to achieve rather than a realistically attainable state. But even if based on a more modest and realistic definition, a right to health and a right to health care are distinctly different ideas. The "right to health care" is a meaningful and understandable social and economic right, despite the repeated refusal by legislators in the United States to establish any basis for its fulfillment in the public or private sector.

The "right to health," however, is a right that no government can fulfill. At best, governments can take preventive steps to improve the health of the population by providing a clean water supply, cleaning up toxic waste dumps, placing restrictions on industrial polluters, and undertaking other public health measures such as mandating the use of seat belts and motorcycle helmets and ensuring an effective system for regulating the manufacture and sale of drugs. Although extreme libertarians argue that requiring motorists to use seat belts and cyclists to wear helmets is an infringement of individual liberty, this is a good example of a social good that arguably outweighs an individual right. But to say that the right to health is a *human* right implies that governments are in violation of this basic human right when their citizens fail to achieve a healthy condition. No government, however wealthy or magnanimous, could possibly achieve that aspirational goal. People will get sick from a wide variety of causes that governments, public health officials, and doctors cannot now prevent or cure and may never be able to.

Perhaps this is a verbal quibble. What the founders of the journal and the many contributors strive to do is to forge a link between the public health community and the efforts of human rights groups. As one contributor says: "If the right to life is the most basic of all human rights, it follows that the right to health and health care are fundamental rights. To die because you are denied medicine, clean water or adequate nutrition is just as much a violation of your right to life as it is to die from a death squad bullet."[38] This is a reminder of the traditional locus of human rights concerns: actions by the state that unjustly deprive citizens of life or liberty.

The principles stated in the Constitution of the WHO include a central claim about rights: "The enjoyment of the highest attainable standard of health is one of the fundamental rights of every human being without distinction of race, religion, political belief, economic or social condition." The WHO Constitution also states that governments bear a responsibility for the health of their people. If the existence of a right establishes a corresponding obligation to fulfill that right, this governmental responsibility can be viewed as embodying a corresponding *duty* implied by the stated fundamental *right* of every human being to the highest attainable standard of health. This would encompass both public health obligations on the part of governments and also an obligation to ensure universal access to medical services. A key question nevertheless remains: Are the *fundamental* rights articulated in the WHO Constitution to be construed as *human* rights? And which specific rights related to medicine and health should properly fall within this scope?

Jonathan Mann, the founder and first editor of the journal *Health and Human Rights*, was killed in a tragic airplane crash in September 1998. Mann was a leading champion of health as a human right and led the world in the struggle against AIDS. At a meeting of the Presidential Advisory Council on HIV/AIDS, Mann said that the U.S. government's failure to proceed to trials of an HIV/AIDS vaccine is a human rights violation. He added: "The ethical problem today in AIDS vaccine development is not in proceeding to trials, but in failing to proceed to trials."[39] It is an ironic twist that failure to carry out research involving human subjects should now be charged with being a human rights violation, given that the conduct of past experiments, such as the infamous Tuskegee study, have led to similar allegations of violations of human rights.

Mann's contention that failure to embark on HIV vaccine trials is a human rights violation sounds a clarion call to move ahead. It is more a political statement than an ethical judgment. To criticize the slow progress on AIDS vaccines as a culpable error of omission may well be an ethically sound judgment. But in calling that omission a violation of human rights, Mann stretched the concept of human rights to its limits. This is because of the virtual impossibility of identifying the individuals whose rights are presumptively violated. It cannot be people living with AIDS because a vaccine would not be a treatment and could do nothing to prevent their having become infected. The bearers of this alleged right could only be those individuals who will become HIV infected but would not have done so if an effective vaccine existed and they had been vaccinated. To be practically useful, claims that charge human rights violations must be able to identify the particular individuals, or the class of individuals, whose rights are being violated. But it is impossible to know who will become HIV positive through lack of an effective AIDS vaccine, who will become HIV positive even if a somewhat effective vaccine is developed, and whom to charge with violating the human rights of those possible future people.

Mann's greatest contributions lay in his arguments contending that health and human rights go hand in hand. He argued persuasively that in the modern world public health officials have, for the first time, two fundamental responsibilities: to protect and promote public health and to protect and promote human rights.[40] Among the human rights Mann addressed are the following: the right not to be tortured or imprisoned under inhumane conditions; the right of HIV-infected people and people with AIDS not to be discriminated against in employment, education, or ability to marry and travel; the right to information, to assembly, or to association; and reproductive rights related to reproductive health. This is truly a mixed bag of rights. The "right not to be tortured or imprisoned under inhumane conditions" lies in the classic category of human rights that people possess against the power and authority of the state. This is as uncontroversial a human right as any.

As we go down the list, however, other alleged human rights may be less evident until we examine the various international instruments in which human rights principles are set forth. The right of people with HIV/AIDS not to be discriminated against is one that some states within the United States and some national governments have embodied in law. It would, in those places, be a violation of the civil laws and of individuals' civil rights to discriminate against them in those ways. In many parts of the world, legal protection of people with HIV/AIDS is entirely lacking, and discrimination persists in many walks of everyday life, including access to medical treatment. Efforts have begun on an international level to adopt guidelines on HIV/AIDS and human rights. For example, a set of guidelines on HIV/AIDS and Human Rights was the product of the Second International Consultation on HIV/AIDS and Human Rights held in Geneva in 1996.[41] The intended users of the guidelines adopted in this forum are legislators and government policy makers.

This international document concerning human rights and AIDS, like the other existing international instruments, includes a wide array of human rights principles.[42] These include the right to life, the right to the highest attainable standard of physical and mental health, the right to liberty and security of the person, the right to privacy, the right to freely receive and impart information, the right to marry and found a family, and the right to an adequate standard of living. We do not have to look at the poorest countries of the world to see that if these international principles of human rights are taken seriously, many human rights are regularly and systematically violated every day. Examples can be found in the United States and other wealthy, industrialized countries. Yet it remains true that most of the human rights in these international instruments are stated in very general terms and consequently require careful interpretation in the various circumstances in which they are to be applied. In this respect, claims about human rights resemble fundamental ethical principles.

Women's Rights and Reproductive Rights as Human Rights

A leading scholar of international law and human rights, Rebecca Cook, reports that international human rights law has not been applied effectively to the disadvantages and injustices experienced by women. Cook contends that in this sense respect for human rights fails to be "universal."[43] She reports the bad news that most governments have fallen far short of ensuring reproductive self-determination for women, but also the good news that some progress is being made in putting the "universal" into reproductive rights as human rights. This observation calls attention to the critical distinction between human rights as a *moral category* that is universally applicable and *respect for* human rights, a factual state of affairs that is far from universal.

International human rights treaties, especially the Convention on the Elimination of All Forms of Discrimination against Women (also known as the Women's Convention), impose at least these obligations on governments: Governments must ensure that women are free from all forms of discrimination, that they are granted the right to liberty and security, and that they have access to health care and the benefits of scientific progress. Taken together, these separate rights under international law converge into a composite right of reproductive self-determination, also known as the right to regulate one's fertility.[44]

Some obvious examples of reproductive rights are the traditional negative rights that mandate freedom from governmental interference in individuals' and couples' procreative activities. An example cited earlier is the Peruvian government's campaign to sterilize women. Ironically, the opposite approach to sterilization can also be found: Laws that prohibit voluntary sterilization are still on the books in Brazil and other countries where Roman Catholicism exerts a strong influence on the legislature. Laws that mandate sterilization of mentally handicapped individuals have been promulgated in China. All such laws or governmental policies interfere with the reproductive freedom of individuals and are therefore in violation of the international covenants that include as human rights the right to liberty, the right to found a family, and the right to determine the number and spacing of one's children.

Whether the leading international human rights instruments can be interpreted to permit legal abortions is, of course, a matter of overwhelming controversy. Women's health advocates the world over argue that at least the following human rights stated in various conventions and covenants mandate noninterference by the state in women's decisions to remain pregnant or to terminate a pregnancy: the right to liberty and security of person, the right to privacy, and especially principle 8 of the ICPD Programme of Action—"all couples and individuals have the basic right to decide freely and responsibly the number and spacing of their children and to have the information, education, and means to do so."[45] But because abortion remains as contentious a matter in the international arena as it is within U.S. politics, governments in Latin America and in Africa, spurred on by the Vatican, as well as by religious and political leaders in their own countries, continue to hold abortion to be a criminal offense rather than a human right.

In defense of the classic catalogue of human rights—individual freedom from oppression by the state and imprisonment for opposition to the government in power—Pope John Paul II has been one of the staunchest proponents. In a visit to Nigeria in 1998 the Pope urged Nigerians to make efforts to guarantee human rights and freedoms. In particular, he called on the then head of state in Nigeria, a military strongman, to release political prisoners.[46] He made a similar plea in a visit to Cuba, following which Fidel Castro ordered the release of political prisoners. Yet the Pope has refused to recognize reproductive rights as a legitimate class of rights because that includes the right to information about contraceptives and access to family planning services, as well as abortion, all of which are forbidden by Catholic Church dogma. This is a perfect example of the difficulty of reaching universal agreement on exactly what counts as a human right, in spite of the broad enunciation of human rights in the numerous international instruments to which many nations have subscribed.

In the discussion of female genital mutilation in Chapter 3, I promised to return to that topic in the context of human rights. It is clear from the various human rights principles described in this chapter that female genital mutilation violates several different statements found in international declarations and conventions. Yet even opponents of female genital mutilation caution critics from outside the countries where it is practiced to avoid calling it a violation of human rights. I attended a meeting in Nigeria in which everyone present concurred that this harmful practice must be eradicated, and, unlike the North American anthropologists cited in Chapter 3, none of the Nigerians at the meeting objected to the word *eradication*. A discussion ensued on whether it is a basic human right of women not to have their genitals cut. Because political torture is (almost) universally acknowledged to violate human rights, I characterized female genital mutilation as violating a fundamental human right of women on grounds that it is a form of "ritual torture." An American pediatrician working in Nigeria cautioned me not to use the word *torture* when it is not the *intent* of parents to commit torture by putting their female infants and children in the hands of traditional healers who perform the cutting. She said it is not a good strategy to use in trying to eradicate the ritual practice of female genital mutilation, adding that the situation is similar to describing as "child abuse" the parental offering of young daughters into prostitution in exchange for money. The intent of the parents is not to subject children to pain, suffering, or abuse, the pediatrician said. These families are desperate for money, and that is their motive in placing their young daughters in prostitution.

We need to distinguish two different points in this objection to the use of value-laden language. The first is whether the meaning of condemnatory language is determined by the intentions of the people who engage in or subscribe to the cultural practice or ritual. The second is the pragmatic consideration of what is the best strategy for success in bringing about change. To the first point I have an old philosophical reply: Motives and intentions have everything to do with the moral character of people, but are usually irrelevant to a judgment of the morality of actions.

As to the second point—a political strategy for eradicating female genital mutilation—I can see the importance of not calling it an act of torture, which would make it a human rights violation, when parents are simply following a widely practiced cultural rite. However, from the point of view of an ethical assessment of such practices, the analogy with torture is arguably still appropriate. The consequences for the individuals subjected to female genital mutilation are identical to harms that would be inflicted on female infants, girls, or women by anyone who had the *intention* of committing torture by this means. One anthropologist, going against the predominant stream, made the unequivocal judgment: "When a young girl is infibulated, on a dirty mat by a nonmedical woman with an old razor, then sewn up with acacia thorns, all without the use of anesthesia, this should be considered a form of torture and a human rights violation."[47] This anthropologist makes the further observation that traditional societies in which such rituals have long been practiced are now undergoing change. She proffers the reasonable hypothesis that resistance to the introduction of human rights in these societies is an attempt by those in power to hold on to what is left of the older community structure.[48]

If agents for a repressive authoritarian government cut the genitals of women prisoners, the intention would be different, but the results for the women's health and sexuality would be identical. The fact that parents and traditional birth attendants do not intend to commit acts of torture is relevant to a judgment of their moral character and could disqualify as inappropriate the label of *torture*. But the intention of a moral agent is not the only factor relevant to making an ethical evaluation of an act that predictably results in excruciating pain, short-term and long-term health effects, and death from shock or hemorrhage.

Although the distinction between making moral judgments of people and evaluating the actions they perform may appear to be an abstract point of ethical theory, I believe it is critically important for determining which cultural practices should properly be viewed as violations of human rights. What makes certain actions violations of human rights is the nature of the acts and their consequences. It is important, therefore, to acknowledge the difference between a political strategy to eradicate female genital mutilation and an ethical analysis of why it should be construed as a violation of a fundamental human right. It is a traditional ritual, the aim of which is to subjugate women by restricting their opportunity or ability to stray from culturally prescribed sexual rules. Even if the "genital surgeries" were carried out by physicians in hospitals, under the most hygienic conditions, they would still mutilate women's bodies with the avowed purpose of keeping them sexually chaste before marriage and abating their interest in or ability to enjoy sex after marriage.

Other traditions that appear to the outside world to involve gross violations of human rights are maintained in different societies. A newspaper article recounted the stories of women in Kenya who were beaten by their husbands with wooden clubs.[49] Domestic violence is a clear violation of "the right to security of the person," and some have argued that violence against women can be characterized as torture.[50] One Kenyan woman who had to be carried to the hospital after one such episode decided to take her husband to court. As a result of her legal action, the woman was made an outcast in her tribe, the Masai. "Women are very angry with me," the woman said, because "it is unheard of in Masailand to put your husband in jail."[51]

There is a law in Kenya against wife beating, but the tradition remains prevalent and is even condoned. An advocacy group in Kenya conducted a survey revealing that 70% of the people interviewed said they knew neighbors who beat their wives. Almost 60% blamed women for the beatings, and only 51% said the men should be punished. Only a small majority of those interviewed favored punishment, yet, despite the prevalence of wife beating, at least some strong opposition to the tradition is evident. The illegality of the practice is evidence that lawmakers have determined that wife-beating is unacceptable, but the reluctance of women to seek legal redress leads to poor enforcement. It is not sufficient for the protection of women's rights merely to have laws on the books. That such laws have been enacted is a reminder that cultural traditions are not static and that people who live in countries where harmful traditions remain are by no means unanimous in support of those traditions.

Human Rights and Ethical Relativism

If human rights is a meaningful concept, and if there are any human rights, then normative ethical relativism must be false. Human rights are, by definition, rights that belong to all people, wherever they may dwell and whatever may be the political system or the cultural traditions of their country or region of the world. The doctrine of normative ethical relativism holds that all moral norms and rules derive from specific cultures. It therefore must deny that there are any universal ethical standards that are (or ought to be) binding on cultural groups or nations despite their ignorance or rejection of those standards. Because human rights embody one such set of universal ethical standards, to remain consistent the ethical relativist must deny that there are any human rights.

To be sure, even if we grant the existence of universal human rights, controversial areas remain. One controversy is whether the category of human rights must be confined to the rights people have against the government or whether the private sphere also includes rights that deserve to be called *human* rights. The right of women not to be beaten by their husbands is an example of a right once thought to exist only in the "private" sphere of the family, immune from state interference. The feminist movement in the United States and internationally has done much to obliterate this traditional distinction between what is public and what is private, thereby opening the door to prosecution of men who batter or rape their wives. If violence within the family becomes a matter of concern to the state, then the family is no longer a sacrosanct preserve of patriarchy. In some countries even today, a man who kills his wife after catching her in bed with another man can be exonerated from the charge of murder. I asked participants in a conference in Brazil whether this is the case in their country. The reply was that if the woman is discovered, her husband can kill her with impunity. Although this is not, strictly speaking, a legitimate legal defense, it is accepted as "customary." When husbands are granted freedom to do whatever they wish to their wives in the "private sphere" of the family, that is a denial of the human rights of women to safety and security of person.

Human rights are rights that people have no matter who may seek to violate them. It does not matter if it is an official of the state who tortures and murders a political prisoner or a midwife who cuts a screaming adolescent's genitals while she is being held down by four other people. It does not matter if it is the military in wartime that makes sexual slaves of captive women or a poverty-stricken peasant who sells his 13-year-old daughter into sexual slavery. All are violations of human rights, as they contravene one or more of the prohibitions enumerated in the international human rights instruments.

Probably the most controversial question remaining is whether positive rights share the status of being human rights with the less controversial negative rights. Although I cannot argue for this thesis here, I contend that some positive rights should occupy the status of human rights. An example is the right to an adequate standard of health care, a standard that (unfortunately) is relative in a different sense of the term. The adequacy of health care and medical services has to be relativized to individual countries and the resources they are able to muster. Poor countries have neither the financial nor the human resources to provide a level of health care that would be considered adequate in an economically developed country. But a wealthy country like the United States is in violation of the human right to an adequate standard of health care by failing to provide for a system that makes such care available to all its inhabitants. Still, a right to health care is not the same as a positive right to health, and the latter concept remains problematic as a human rights claim.

If we grant the legitimacy of the category of human rights—the debates over various particulars notwithstanding—then one further controversial question should be addressed. That is whether the concept of "moral progress" is meaningful and appropriate. Although posing that question once again raises the specter of ethical imperialism, we cannot ignore the movement of history that has resulted in a growing recognition of rights that belong to all people, wherever they may live, and whatever may be their racial, ethnic, religious, or economic background.

Notes

1. Jay Katz, "Human Experimentation and Human Rights," *Saint Louis University Law Journal*, Vol. 38, No. 1 (1993), pp. 7–54.

2. Katz, p. 52.

3. Council of Europe, Directorate of Legal Affairs, "Convention for the Protection of Human Rights and Dignity of the Human Being with Regard to the Application of Biology and Medicine: Convention on Human Rights and Bioethics" (Strasbourg: Council of Europe, June 6, 1996).

4. Council of Europe, Convention, p. 2.

5. David Shapiro, "Think Before You Squawk," *New Scientist*, August 2, 1997.

6. Rebecca J. Cook, *Human Rights in Relation to Women's Health* (Geneva: World Health Organization, 1993).

7. Lawrence O. Gostin and Zita Lazzarini, *Human Rights and Public Health in the AIDS Pandemic* (New York: Oxford University Press, 1997).

8. Interview with Mercy Fabros, September 1992, during my visit to the Philippines as part of my Ford Foundation project.

9. Ren-Zong Qui, "What Has Bioethics To Offer the Developing Countries?" *Bioethics*, Vol. 7, No. 2/3 (1993), p. 118.

10. Patricia A. Marshall, "Anthropology and Bioethics," *Medical Anthropology Quarterly* Vol. 6, No. 1, p. 54.

11. Physicians in India reported this in my visit there in March 1994 as part of my Ford Foundation project.

12. This was reported to me in my Ford Foundation visit to Bangladesh in April 1994.

13. This was described to me during my Ford Foundation project visit to Mexico in February 1993.

14. Maurice Cranston, "Are There Any Human Rights?" *Daedalus*, Vol. 112, No. 4 (1983), p. 11.

15. Cranston, p. 1.

16. Alison T. Slack, "Female Circumcision: A Critical Appraisal," *Human Rights Quarterly* Vol. 10 (1988), p. 473.

17. "Statement on Human Rights," *American Anthropologist*, Vol. 49, No. 4 (1947), p. 542.

18. Adamantia Pollis and Peter Schwab, "Human Rights: A Western Construct with Limited Applicability," (eds.) Adamantia Pollis and Peter Schwab, *Human Rights: Cultural and Ideological Perspectives* (New York: Praeger Publishers, 1979), p. 1.

19. Universal Declaration of Human Rights, adopted December 10, 1948; G.A. Res. 217A (III), U.N. Doc. A/810 (1948).

20. Cranston, p. 12.

21. Cranston, pp. 12–13.

22. Christopher Clausen, "Welcome to Postculturalism," *The Key Reporter*, Vol. 62, No. 1 (1996), p. 3.

23. Elaine Sciolino, "U.S. Rejects Notion that Human Rights Vary with Culture," *New York Times* (June 15, 1993), p. A1.

24. Steven Erlanger, "Malaysia's Conspiracy Theory Draws Criticism from Albright," *New York Times* (July 29, 1997), p. A8.

25. Mab Huang, "Human Rights in a Revolutionary Society: The Case of the People's Republic of China" (eds.) Adamantia Pollis and Peter Schwab, *Human Rights: Cultural and Ideological Perspectives* (New York: Praeger Publishers, 1979), p. 63.

26. Merle Goldman, "Human Rights in the People's Republic of China," *Daedalus*, Vol. 112, No. 4 (1983), p. 111.

27. Xiaorong Li, "Asian Values' and the University of Human Rights," *Report from the Institute for Philosophy & Public Policy*, Vol. 16, No. 2 (1996), pp. 18–23.

28. Li, p. 20.

29. Li, p. 21.

30. Seth Faison, "China Turns the Tables, Faulting U.S. on Rights," *New York Times* (March 5, 1997), p. A8.

31. Faison, p. A8.

32. Xiaorong Li, "A Question of Priorities: Human Rights, Development, and 'Asian Values,'" *Report from the Institute for Philosophy & Public Policy*, Vol. 18, Nos. 1, 2 (1998), pp. 7–12.

33. Li, p. 7.

34. Li, p. 9.

35. Esther B. Fein, "Calling Infertility a Disease, Couples Battle with Insurers," *New York Times* (February 22, 1998), p. 34.

36. Gaby Ore Aguilar, "Letter to the Editor," *New York Times* (February 21, 1998), p. A10.

37. John F. Lauerman, "Welcome to *Health and Human Rights*," *Health and Human Rights*, Vol. 1, No. 1 (1994), p. 3.

38. Laurie S. Wiseberg, "The Opening of a Dialogue," *Health and Human Rights*, Vol. 2, No. 2 (1995), p. 121.

39. Jonathan Mann, presentation before PACHA, "Failure To Proceed to AIDS Vaccine Trials is a Human Rights Violation," from an NCIH Global AIDS Program press release on the World Wide Web, 15 March 1998.

40. Jonathan M. Mann, "Medicine and Public Health, Ethics and Human Rights," *Hastings Center Report*, Vol. 27, No. 3 (1997), p. 9.

41. Commission on Human Rights, Economic and Social Council, United Nations: Second International Consultation on HIV/AIDS and Human Rights, January 10, 1997.

42. These instruments include but are not limited to the Universal Declaration of Human Rights; the International Covenants on Economic, Social and Cultural Rights and on Civil and Political Rights; the Convention of the Elimination of All Forms of Discrimination against Women; the Convention on the Rights of the Child.

43. Rebecca Cook, "Women's International Human Rights Law: The Way Forward," *Human Rights Quarterly* Vol. 15 (993), p. 231.

44. Rebecca Cook, "Putting the 'Universal' into Human Rights," *Populi* Vol. 21, No. 7 (1994), pp. 15–16.

45. Programme of Action of the United Nations International Conference on Population and Development, ICPD Secretariat, U.N. Doc. A/CONF.171/13 (1994).

46. "Pope, in Nigeria, Appeals for Human Rights" (Reuters), *New York Times* (March 22, 1998), p. 6.

47. Slack, p. 466.

48. Slack, p. 475.

49. "Kenyan Tradition Confronted: A Beaten Wife Goes to Court," (AP), *New York Times* (October 31, 1997), p. A5.

50. Cook. pp. 248–250.

51. "Kenyan Tradition Confronted: A Beaten Wife Goes to Court."

10

Moral
Progress
and
Ethical
Universals

DEBATES about the meaning of *moral progress*[1] and whether human history demonstrates such progress are linked to the controversy surrounding ethical relativism. Earlier in this century, anthropologists who deplored racism in the United States, as evidenced in U.S. immigration laws, sought to combat racism through their anthropological studies. This mixture of antiracist values with cultural relativism has remained a powerful force up to the present day. As noted in Chapter 2, the nineteenth century view of "cultural evolutionism" was a theory describing the progression of human societies in hierarchical stages from "primitive" or "savage" (represented by tribal, nonliterate societies) to a more "progressed" form of culture (represented by Western civilization). Cultural relativism was introduced in part to combat these racist, hierarchical Eurocentric ideas of progress.[2]

However, to adopt a moral stance against racism and at the same time to espouse ethical relativism embodies a contradiction. The judgment that racism is wrong is an ethical judgment, one that antiracists believe has universal moral validity. Not only is it wrong for white Americans to discriminate against black Americans, and for white Canadians to discriminate against indigenous people; it is also wrong for Hutus to seek to wipe out Tutsis, for Japanese to discriminate against Koreans in their midst, and for Hindus to maintain a system that discriminates hierarchically according to the caste into which people are born. Can an ethical relativist consistently reject the appropriateness of making moral judgments about other cultures and at the same time maintain that racism practiced in those cultures is wrong?

It would be hard to deny that today's moral condemnation of racism, wherever it may exist, is an example of moral progress. Laws designed to eliminate—or, perhaps more realistically, minimize—racial discrimination in employment, education, and housing constitute an example of moral progress in public policy. The introduction of the language of human rights into the global conversation, along with the various charges, defenses, and countercharges of human rights violations, represents another ethical advance over earlier eras. But the concept of moral progress can only be understood against a backdrop of ethical universals. In the absence of a foundation built on general ethical principles, claims that moral progress has occurred would be meaningless or indefensible.

The concept of moral progress, as I will argue here, is a social concept: It applies only to events, institutions, and social practices in countries, cultures, societies, eras, or periods in history, not to individual persons or personal moral behavior. The idea of moral progress is relational, that is, it expresses a relation of moral comparison between two or more different elements (e.g., cultures, societies, historical eras). I offer two fundamental principles to serve as criteria for judging moral progress. These principles are hardly novel, as their roots lie in prominent theories of philosophical ethics. First is "the principle of humaneness": One culture, society, or historical era exhibits a higher degree of moral progress than another if the first shows more sensitivity to (less tolerance of) the pain and suffering of human beings than does the second, as expressed in the laws, customs, institutions, and practices of the respective societies or eras.[3] This principle has its basis in utilitarian moral philosophy. Second is "the principle of humanity": One culture, society, or era exhibits a higher degree of moral progress than another if the first shows more recognition of the equal worth and basic autonomy of every human being than does the second, as expressed in the laws, customs, institutions, and practices of the respective societies or eras. This principle is rooted in the Kantian philosophical tradition.

The principle of humaneness reflects the core meaning of the term *humane*, which connotes compassion, sympathy, and consideration for the suffering of other human beings (as well as sentient animal life). The principle of humanity captures the sense of the term *humanity* as referring to the totality of attributes that distinguish humans from other creatures or as denoting the "essential" human quality or character. These two principles stem from the two universal attributes of the human species that give rise to morality as an institution—the *sentience* and the *rationality* of persons, the attributes that lie at the core of utilitarian and deontological moral theories. Where these major philosophical theories yield ethical judgments that come into conflict, these will also be the rare instances in which my criteria also come into conflict with one another. But this exactly mirrors our ambivalence in moral sentiments and our uncertainty in moral convictions when we are presented with such examples. As criteria for evaluating moral progress, these two principles do not and cannot resolve disputes that lie at the foundation of ethics. We do not have to reject the significance of respect for autonomy to maintain that the suffering and deprivation of others is cause for concern. And we do not commit ourselves to an oppressive political system if we allow for circumstances in which the welfare of society as a whole calls for relegating individual autonomy to second place.

To avoid misunderstanding, I need to clarify further what I am calling *moral progress*. It should not be understood as a factual description of how people actually behave or have changed their behavior. It is not the rise and fall of crime rates that serve to indicate whether moral progress has occurred, but rather the changes in laws in the direction of greater humaneness and respect for humanity in every person. People, of course, violate the law. Laws prohibit police brutality and citizens express public outrage at its occurrence, but such brutality continues to occur. A moral system, being an ideal of conduct, is based on principles that must be apprehended by reason. But people sometimes act from motives that are contrary to reason and common sense.

The concept of moral progress unpacks into these two principles— "humaneness" and "humanity"—so we need to show how these principles are supposed to work as criteria for judgments of moral progress. The most plausible answer is that satisfying either one of these principles is sufficient to make the judgment that moral progress exists or has taken place. However, if both principles are satisfied, there is a greater degree of moral progress than if only one principle is exemplified in any given judgement that moral progress has occurred. Admittedly, most of the key terms in the principles of humaneness and humanity are vague or denote qualities that are hard to measure, such as "sensitivity to" or "tolerance of" pain and suffering and "recognition of the universal worth or basic autonomy" of every human being. But even if the terms in which these two principles are couched are rather vague, the signs by which we know them in social and political life are clear and unmistakable. Behavioral and contextual evidence, as well as laws and rules that govern behavior, are the signs.

When laws prohibit "cruel and unusual punishment" it is a sign of moral progress over earlier eras when the hands of thieves were cut off for stealing and when criminals were tortured on racks or pilloried in public. If the objection is made that some religious dictates still mandate amputation of the hands of thieves, two different replies are possible. The first is that religious mandates or practices should not be exceptions to judgments of moral progress. Proposed as universal principles, the criteria for judging moral progress apply to religious practices as well as to secular actions. Thus cutting off the hands of thieves is a morally regressive form of punishment compared with other sanctions.

The second, quite different reply is that religion should be viewed as standing higher than or apart from the moral law, with each religion providing moral laws unto itself. The latter reply makes a claim for religious exceptionalism and is therefore simply another version of ethical relativism. I see no good reason why religious mandates and practices should be immune from ethical judgments any more than cultural practices or traditions. Although it is true that religious beliefs are matters of faith rather than observation and reason, that does not place religious practices beyond the pale of moral judgment. It is a different question entirely whether outsiders may employ means to change the practices that are accepted by religious adherents but that violate fundamental ethical principles.

The principle of humaneness is couched in terms of levels of tolerance for conditions of pain and suffering. Despite the vagueness of this idea, levels of tolerance are expressed in laws and accepted practices, as well as in public debates among policy makers and citizens. It is clear when positive steps are taken to alleviate social pain and suffering through political action and changes in laws. A further indicator of moral progress is the sorts of arguments given on behalf of these changes.

Another objection from religion enters the picture: that suffering is ennobling. Some religions extol suffering, for example, the early Christian view that bodily suffering and punishments imposed on the body are a means of reaching toward Christ.[4] Another Judeo-Christian religious viewpoint takes suffering to be a punishment by God for individual or group actions or sins, and in that sense, a form of divine retributive justice. Monks in various religions live a life of self-abnegation that, even if not de-

signed to produce manifest suffering, certainly amounts to a denial of pleasure. None of these religious beliefs or behaviors has any bearing on the
principle of humaneness as a measure of moral progress. People are free
to follow what they take to be divine commands and impose suffering
on themselves. But when a powerful group in society imposes suffering
on others, or when the state chooses to ignore the suffering of its members
by failing to take workable steps to remedy that suffering, the religious
dictate that "suffering is ennobling" is irrelevant. As an ethical criterion
for evaluating social and governmental concern for human suffering,
the principle of humaneness stands apart from any particular religious
doctrine.

It is also clear by a range of public criteria when one culture or historical era exhibits greater respect for the equal worth and basic autonomy
of human beings. Fair employment legislation, equal rights amendments,
judicial decisions mandating school desegregation, and rulings prohibiting discrimination based on race, sex, or disability—all these exemplify
a conscious effort in society to ensure that all citizens enjoy rights formerly
guaranteed to an elite or to white people or men only. To the degree that
laws, social practices, and ethical beliefs change in the direction of greater
recognition of the equal worth and respect for all individuals, to that extent
moral progress takes place. Social reformers, judges, legislators, moral theorists, and advocacy groups often justify their proposed changes or those
already wrought by appealing to the ethical ideas embodied in these two
principles.

The Individual Versus the "Common Good"

At this point , a well-known and well-worn objection inevitably arises. It is
that autonomy is a peculiarly Western idea deriving from the importance
Western societies accord to the individual. This familiar objection continues: Other cultures place greater value on the community as a whole, on
the family unit more than on its individual members. According to this objection, the principle of humanity, focusing as it does on the worth of each
individual and on respect for each individual's basic autonomy, is pecu-

liarly Eurocentric. It will be said that to elevate it to the level of a universal ethical principle is yet another instance of ethical imperialism.

It is true that the principle of humanity, as I have defined it here, calls for universal respect for autonomy. However, nothing in the principle says how the rights of the individual and the needs of society ought to be balanced in cases where they come into conflict. The principle does not impose an absolute priority of the individual over other societal units and considerations. Critics of the principle of respect for autonomy often make this error: They confuse its universal applicability with the mistaken idea that it is absolute. No Western or European nation grants to individuals rights that have absolute priority over the needs of the community as a whole. What the principle does require is recognition by governments and other powerful authorities that individuals have basic rights to liberty and self-determination.

In the quest to avoid ethical imperialism and at the same time to arrive at an international, multicultural bioethics, one ethicist urges a turning away from the narrow constraints of autonomy and individual rights.[5] David Thomasma asks: "Could bioethics worldwide be based on some other principle than patient rights?"[6] In his generally thoughtful essay, Thomasma nevertheless buys into the widely believed and oft-stated dogma that Western bioethics is preoccupied with autonomy and self-determination. It is true, of course, that discussions of the doctor–patient relationship have focused on patients' right to autonomy against the traditional paternalism of doctors. As I discussed in Chapter 4, however, other countries have begun to move in the same direction but not because Western ethicists, political leaders, or policy makers have sought to impose their view in a demonstration of ethical imperialism.

Western bioethics has been concerned with a great many other topics besides the rights of patients. The use of appropriate medical technology, the problem of inequitable access to health care, fairness in the distribution of organs for transplantation and other limited resources, placing limits on the commodification of the body and bodily products in surrogacy and the sale of human eggs, gene therapy, germ-line research, and the ethics of genetic enhancement—all these are topics and themes explored in the literature and conferences of Western bioethics.

Thomasma urges that an alternative be sought to autonomy as the basis of human rights and proposes "the common good tradition that has influenced Western thought since Aristotle."[7] In that tradition, "individual good and rights coincide with the community's good."[8] To my knowledge, the Greeks and Romans did not have anything to say about individual rights. Beyond that, what they most certainly did not do is consider the good of *all* individuals to count in their reckoning of the common good.

Plato and Aristotle, the major thinkers of Greek civilization, defended the practice of slavery. Aristotle's defense of this social arrangement was based on his view that some people are "natural slaves" and others are "natural masters." It is undoubtedly true that some people have traits that make them good leaders, while others are better followers. But it does not follow from those observable differences that the former should be ethically permitted to own the latter and treat them like property. Aristotle made numerous sophisticated distinctions in his ethical theory, including distinctions between intentional and unintentional conduct and between voluntary and involuntary conduct, and he gave a finely tuned account of human virtues. It seems fair to say that Aristotle and others of his time had a moral blind spot when it came to the enslavement of persons. Based on the sophistication of his own ethical theory, he ought to have seen that it is not ethically permissible for human beings to own other human beings like inanimate property. But that social arrangement was believed to contribute to the good of the community, so it could be justified on those grounds.

Despite Thomasma's valiant effort and thoughtful reflections, it is impossible to establish a basis of human rights in the "common good tradition." This is because the "common good" is the good of the whole society or community, and human rights can only be ascribed to individuals. It does not follow, however, that individual rights always trump the interests of the community. What does follow is that the particular rights properly termed *human rights* may be overridden only in extreme and extenuating circumstances. The good for the society in times of war, famine, natural disaster, plague, and other ills can justify the abridgment of certain individual rights, including fundamental rights like liberty. To acknowledge the existence and defend the importance of individual rights does not rule out the circumstances in which they may legitimately be abridged or over-ridden in the interest of the larger community.

Cross-Cultural Ethical Judgments

How can the concept of moral progress be used in making cross-cultural ethical judgments? The principles of humaneness and humanity, like any general ethical principle, require interpretation in light of particular facts and circumstances. Also like other general ethical principles, they cannot be applied "deductively," as critics of the use of principles mistakenly suppose an appeal to principles requires. Nevertheless, application of these principles yields some uncontroversial conclusions. For example, the principle of humanity demands recognition of the worth of women equal to that of men and respect for women's capacity and authority to make decisions. It yields the judgment that societies or cultures where women are the property of men, where they may not visit a doctor without their husbands' permission, where they may not use birth control without their husbands' authorization, where they may be beaten by their husbands for going to the movies without permission—these societies or cultures are less morally progressed in this regard than those that recognize women's right to liberty and self-determination equal to that of men.

By way of further illustration, I offer three brief examples of existing cultural practices that can be judged to exhibit a lower level of moral progress than those in societies where such practices are forbidden by law or rejected by ethical norms. The first is the treatment of widows according to Hindu custom in parts of India, described more fully in Chapter 2; the second is the treatment of women by the militant Islamic Taliban movement in Afghanistan; and the third is the continued existence of human slavery in Mauritania.

Recall that in parts of India, Hindu brides marry into their husbands' families and, when the husband dies, the widow is left entirely dependent on her in-laws. If she is young, she may be forced to work as an unpaid servant for her mother-in-law for decades to come. Many widows are thrown out of the house, and others leave on their own accord, compelling them to resort to begging or prostitution. Although inheritance laws in modern India grant widows rights to a share of their husbands' property, tradition outweighs everything and the laws are ignored.[9] In regard to these modern inheritance laws, India demonstrates moral progress over earlier eras. But with respect to adherence to tradition, the cultural groups that treat widows abominably are less morally progressed than the majority in India who have moved beyond what is mandated in ancient Hindu texts.

The plight of women in Afghanistan today is arguably worse than that of the Indian widows, in part because the Taliban strictures apply to all women and in part because the prohibitions are so pervasive. When the Taliban movement took over the government by force in 1996, it decreed that women could no longer work outside the home, they must cover themselves from head to toe when they venture outside the home, and girls are prohibited from attending school.[10] The consequences are not only the virtual imprisonment of Afghanistan women in their own homes, but also a distinct shortage of teachers and nurses in the country, occupations normally filled by women. Although exceptions to this universal repression of women can be found, they are relatively few.

In Mauritania today, an estimated 90,000 black people serve as slaves to the Arabs who rule the country.[11] Although the government says it has abolished slavery, the existence of a population of hard laborers owned as property is documented. The institution of slavery is apparently accepted by the slaves as well as their owners, and there is no rebellion, no need to chain the slaves to keep them from running away, and the slaves themselves have no idea that any other options could exist for them. In fact, an ordinance in 1980 by the then president of Mauritania freed the slaves, but without making slave ownership illegal. No one has informed the slaves that they are legally emancipated. Some do succeed in leaving their bondage, and many of those fail to eke out a meager existence, so they return to slavery. The apparent acceptance of their lot and absence of any rebellion on the part of these slaves does not show that their enslavement can be ethically justified. People need not *feel* degraded in order to *be* degraded by a social practice.

A detailed ethical analysis is hardly necessary to show that treating women whose husbands have died as indentured servants or, alternatively, as outcasts fails to respect their worth as human beings. No additional facts are needed to demonstrate that women in Afghanistan, having been denied education and freedom of movement, are decreed by law to occupy an oppressed and demeaning status. As for the continued practice of sanctioned slavery in the Islamic Republic of Mauritania, it is safe to conclude that few institutions in the history of humankind have been as degrading as the treatment of people as property. It is undeniable that these three cultures are less morally progressed than most others in today's world.

To judge those societies as less morally progressed is not to manifest ethical imperialism. People within oppressive societies seek social and legal reforms, not because they want to emulate the West but because they judge their own culture to have serious moral flaws. Women and men in Nigeria, Egypt, and other African countries who are working to eradicate the ritual of female genital mutilation are implicitly comparing their own culture, in which the rite is practiced, with other parts of the world in which it is not. When they base the need for reform on the personal harms and public health consequences to women of female genital mutilation, they are appealing to the principle of humaneness. They believe that large numbers of women and girls in their society would have less pain and suffering if this practice were eliminated. If they base the need for reform on the circumstance that most women (including female infants and young girls) who undergo the procedure do not do so voluntarily, they are implicitly appealing to the principle of humanity, recognizing the autonomy and worth of individual women. Inherent in any reform movement, be it social, political, or moral, is a comparison between what does exist and what ought to exist. If there is ethical content to the reform movement, then its supporters believe that moral progress will occur if the reforms can successfully be brought about.

The awakening in many parts of the world that research subjects and patients have rights may have had its origins in North America, but that does not mean these rights should not be granted to patients and research subjects everywhere. If people have a right not to be used "merely as a means," then voluntary, informed consent to be a research subject is a human right, not simply an artifact of federal regulations in the United States and similar rules in Western Europe. Moral progress has certainly occurred in the research enterprise, allowing us to condemn Tuskegee, Willowbrook, human radiation experiments, and other sorry episodes of exploitation of human subjects in past research in the United States. It follows that people living in countries or cultures where such practices persist today may legitimately call for reforms in order that progress in recognizing the rights of research participants may occur there, as well.

Judgments about moral progress require precision, as the situations that give rise to such judgments are often quite complex. One example is a news report that described a change in the abortion law in Algeria to permit exceptions in the cases of women who were abducted and raped by militant Islamic rebels.[12] The law prohibiting abortions in Algeria previously had no such exceptions. But pressure from women's organizations led to authorization by the Islamic Supreme Council, the highest religious authority in Algeria. The plight of the women who were victims of roving bands of men of the Armed Islamic Group has been doubly severe. A number estimated as well over 2,000 were abducted, raped, and subsequently killed. More than 1,000—possibly as many as or more than 1,600—were raped and let go or escaped. But because of the conservative traditions in the country, many of the families of the women who became pregnant as a result of rape refused to allow them to return home. As these numbers increased, the women's organizations that have helped the women agitated for government action to provide housing and medical care.

This grim episode has elements of moral progress and aspects of moral regress and demonstrates the inhumanity and inhumaneness of this type of conservative cultural tradition. Moral progress is exemplified in the government's and Islamic Supreme Council's willingness to grant exceptions to a restrictive abortion law for women who become pregnant as a result of savage acts of rape by fundamentalist religious militants. It is an act of humaneness by the government to relax the abortion law for women who suffer dishonor in their culture from being forcibly impregnated. *Moral regress* is too weak a term to describe the organized attacks by armed soldiers acting out of religious zeal. Although *savagery* or *brutality* would be a more apt term, *moral regress* characterizes the lapse from Islamic religious ideals in the treatment of women. The holy Qu'ran commands the Muslim man to respect women (albeit particularly in their role as mothers) and to obey the Islamic laws that grant women important rights (rights that are nevertheless unequal to those of men).[13] Abduction, rape, and slaughter of women in the name of Islam is the extreme opposite of what the scriptures mandate.

The refusal by traditional Algerian families to allow women who have been raped and impregnated back into the home is an example of cultural tradition that places the avoidance of shame, humiliation, and dishonor above the humane concerns for family members who have been wronged and harmed. If Western culture is criticized for placing too much value on the autonomous individual and not enough on the family, cultural traditions like this in Algeria can be criticized for their lack of family solidarity where family members are cruelly victimized. Chapter 3 described an analogous situation in which adolescent and pre-adolescent girls are placed into early marriage by their families because of the fear that they might become pregnant before marrying and thus dishonor the family. These are among the societies often exalted for their "family values."

The ethical relativist would say there is no objective way to rank the competing moral values of dishonor to families in traditional cultures, on the one hand, and on the other hand the suffering to women who are made outcasts or who bear the consequences of obstructed labor from undergoing childbirth before they have reached maturity. Avoidance of dishonor to families is their traditional value, concern for the plight of women our modern, Western value. Who is to say which value should take precedence when they come into conflict? The answer is that some moral values are more fundamental than others and, therefore, deserve to be recognized as universal. Middle-level or intermediate values may remain culturally relative.

Although family pride and honor are accorded paramount importance in some traditional cultures, they occupy that status at the expense of the health, the familial embrace, and even sometimes the lives of women and girls, as in the examples just given. Only by devaluing women's lives and health to a status significantly lower than that of family honor can this traditional system be justified. "Respect for family honor" in these cultures is a more important value than the principle "respect for the equal worth of women."

It would be naive and mistaken to maintain that all moral values are equal in weight or importance; so some basis must be found for judging some to be higher than others. That is precisely the intent of human rights declarations and covenants: to place some moral values (the ones articulated in the documents) on a higher plane than others. The Declaration of Human Rights includes the provision in Article 3, "Everyone has the right to life, liberty, and the security of person" and Article 5, "No one shall be subjected to torture or to cruel, inhuman or degrading treatment or punishment." The Declaration makes no mention of any corresponding "rights" to uphold family honor. Human rights, because they are held to be universal moral values, therefore stand higher than values embodied in limited cultural traditions. Societies that recognize and adhere to human rights exhibit greater moral progress than those that place cultural traditions above the mandates of human rights.

What Turns Out To Be Relative?

One philosopher's approach to cultural and ethical relativism was noted briefly in Chapter 2. That was the response of Carl Wellman in answer to the question: What follows from the facts of cultural relativity? "What follows depends in part upon just what turns out to be relative. . . . There are at least ten quite different things of interest to the ethicist that the anthropologist might discover to be relative to culture: mores, social institutions, human nature, acts, goals, value experiences, moral emotions, moral concepts, moral judgments and moral reasoning."[14] The wide array of examples cited in the foregoing chapters suggests that some of the 10 items are quite clearly relative to culture (mores, value experiences, and goals), others appear to rest on cultural universals (human nature, moral emotions), and others require a great deal of interpretation and elucidation (social institutions, moral concepts, moral judgments).

Take, for example, moral concepts. Japanese authorities introduced the idea of "Japanese informed consent" (Chapter 4), and a Chinese scholar distinguished between "the Western principle of autonomy" and "the East Asian principle of autonomy" (Chapter 4). Even the idea that there is a single "Western" concept of autonomy was challenged by the Spanish scholar (Chapter 1) who argued that the term *autonomy* acquired different meanings in the United States and in Europe.

What the Japanese authorities endeavored to do was to preserve some of the paternalistic features of traditional medical practice. It is not the meaning of the concept of informed consent that differs from the Western meaning but, rather, the number and type of requirements imposed by the doctrine of informed consent. On the other hand, the concept of autonomy may well be ambiguous. Its core meaning is "capacity for self-rule," but where the individual self is viewed as inextricably linked with the social unit of the family, a legitimate concept of family autonomy, subsuming the individual, could exist side by side with the starkly individualistic Western concept. As for the idea that there are "Italian ethical principles," that odd cultural entity could readily be dismissed when it turned out that paternalistic features of the 1989 Italian Code of Medical Ethics were eliminated a mere 5 years later.

Even moral emotions could, in some cases, turn out to be culturally relative. Recall the emotions described by a Japanese physician explaining why a prognosis of terminal illness is withheld from patients (Chapter 4). The physicians said that this behavior is rooted in the Japanese ethos in which silent endurance is a virtue. The aim of withholding bad news is not to invoke a dogma of avoiding telling patients the truth, but to make dying easier. Patients want to die as calmly and peacefully as possible, and that goal is more readily achieved if they remain ignorant of their prognosis. But like many observers, that physician pointed to Western influences in his country and a shift toward what he termed a "more ethical emphasis, closer to the Western style of dealing with death." A reminder, once again, that cultures are not static, but evolve constantly both from within and in response to outside influences.

The traditional Navajos hold the belief that thinking and speaking in a negative way can produce the very harms thought or discussed, and so positive thinking is required to maintain health. As described in Chapter 5, this belief causes problems for health professionals seeking to carry out the mandate of the Patient Self-Determination Act and also compromises the ability of physicians to disclose the risks of treatment in an informed

consent discussion with patients. The difference between the Navajo beliefs about causality and those of Western science creates the following apparent dilemma: either respect the Navajo belief system and the ethical
consequences that follow, which leads to a substandard version of informed consent and disclosure; or else adhere to the well-accepted, prevailing dictates of consent and disclosure, thereby risking harm to the Native Americans who hold the traditional beliefs. The first horn of the
dilemma appears to embrace normative ethical relativism, whereas the
second horn looks a lot like ethical imperialism.

We can escape between the horns. My solution to the Navajo conun-
drum lay in an appeal to ethical principles at a more fundamental level
than the middle-level discourse of informed consent. The principle of
beneficence supports the withholding of information about risks of treatment from Navajos who adhere to the traditional belief system, but so, too,
does the principle of respect for autonomy. Navajos holding traditional beliefs can act autonomously only when they are not thinking in a negative
way, so physicians who withhold bad news are not being paternalistic in
the usual sense (acting in what *they* believe is in the patient's best interest).
Instead, they are acting in what the Navajo patients themselves believe is
in their own best interest, and that shows respect for autonomy. A degree of
ethical relativism is undeniably present in the less-than-ideal version of informed consent, and it does admittedly constitute a "lower" standard than
that which is usually appropriate in today's medical practice. However, it
heeds the call for cultural awareness and sensitivity by framing the obligation of disclosure in a way that can be applied in any cultural context:
"Conduct the informed consent discussion in a manner appropriate to the
patient's beliefs and understanding." To relativize informed consent procedures to the cultural background of patients is analogous to relativizing the
discussion to patients' educational level. That is not a pernicious form of
ethical relativism, but is instead an avoidance of mindless rigidity. Procedures can and must be flexible, and that flexibility is still consistent with
adherence to more fundamental ethical principles.

A culturally relative view of rationality was described in Chapter 5.
That view was expressed by the commentators on the case of the Iu Mien
woman who burned her child in a healing ritual. The commentators de-

fended the Mien woman's belief system as entirely rational: "It is well grounded in her culture; it is practiced widely; the reasons for it are widely understood among the Iu Mien; the procedure, from a Mien point of view, works." To place the burning procedure on a par with practices that "work" from the point of view of Western medicine is to adopt a strange conception of rationality. Recall that if the skin does not blister, the Mien belief is that the illness may be related to spiritual causes and a shaman might have to be called; also that the Mien woman said that if the burns are not done in the right place, the baby could become mute or even retarded. Does "rationality" require that we suspend the beliefs of Western medical science about causality and grant equal status to the Mien beliefs?

My conclusion in this case appeals both to the principle of beneficence and also to a conception of justice: To refrain from educating such parents and from exhorting them to alter their traditional practices is unjust, as it exposes immigrant children to health risks that are not borne by children from the majority culture. If "cultural sensitivity" requires this form of inhumane behavior on the part of physicians, it signals a moral regress. And if it justifies giving different medical treatment to children who are unwittingly harmed by their immigrant parents than physicians would provide for children who are victims of intentional child abuse, then a consequence of "cultural sensitivity" is differential treatment based on ethnicity.

Traditional Japanese beliefs about spiritual and bodily unity have consequences for the permissibility of autopsy and for acceptance of the brain death criterion, as we saw in Chapter 6. The acceptability of organ donation in the Philippines relies on the Filipino belief requiring a particular motivation on the part of the organ donor. These beliefs and practices differ from those in the West and are clear instances of cultural diversity. What follows for ethics?

Global Multiculturalism

A definition of *multiculturalism* was quoted in Chapter 5: "a social–intellectual movement that promotes the value of diversity as a core principle

and insists that all cultural groups be treated with respect and as equals."
An underpinning of multiculturalism is the idea of tolerance for the beliefs and practices of subcultures within a larger society, a view often expressed as "the need to be culturally sensitive." In the global community,
the same principle of tolerance is urged, as it is a requirement for cultural
sensitivity. The virtues of toleration and sensitivity surely deserve cultiva-
tion and constant practice. Who among us would defend intolerance and
insensitivity as virtues? Yet the trouble with basing an ethical system on
these, as on other virtues, is that they fail to give clear guidance in the face
of brutal, inhumane, and savage conduct by adherents of cultural traditions and fundamentalist zealots. Virtues are fine, as far as they take us,
but they do not enable us to make moral judgments of poor peasants who
sell their girl children into sexual slavery. "Religious toleration" does not
tell us how to respond to Islamic fundamentalists in Algeria who kidnap,
rape, and murder women, nor does "cultural sensitivity" enlighten us on
how to react to the families who reject the raped women who have man-
aged to survive. Of course, we may remain nonjudgmental in all of these
cases. If ethical relativism is true, we have no choice but to be nonjudgmental.

The exhortation to be "culturally sensitive," like other exhortations to
virtue, provides no tools for ethical justification. The telling of narratives,
however rich and intriguing, can *explain* individual or group conduct, but
can never *justify* a moral judgment about such conduct. Why do we need
to judge in the first place? So we have a basis for determining that our own
moral behavior, as well as that of others, stands in need of improvement.
That is the road to moral progress, improvement in our customs, laws, and
social institutions. Why do we need ethical justification? Without it, moral
judgment would be arbitrary, if not capricious.

Some will say I have not succeeded in meeting the challenge posed
by the world's cultural diversity. That challenge relies on a fundamental
feature of some cultures that would make the principle of humanity inapplicable. The principle is inapplicable to those societies in which the community, rather than the individual, is the basic unit. In such societies individuals have no identity outside the community; their roles are not defined
independently but in virtue of how they contribute to the community. The

individual is not recognized as having any status apart from culturally defined roles — within the family or in relation to the society as a whole. As a result, it is totally meaningless to ascribe rights to individual persons, rights that they may claim against other persons or against the community of which they are a part.

This is a challenge that must be reckoned with. If the description it provides is accurate, it calls for one of two radically different responses. The first is to conclude that such societies demonstrate a very low degree of moral progress because they have not gotten to the point of recognizing individuals as having any value apart from their being cogs in a more important wheel, contributing to the larger group. Individuals are seen as a means merely, if it is at all meaningful to speak of individuals apart from the group. If "respect for persons" is the core interpretation of the principle of humanity, a society that cannot even apply the principle is less morally progressed than societies that recognize the worth of each individual. To draw this conclusion is to open oneself to the classic charge of ethical imperialism.

A second response confronts the challenge by asking for a rich description of the culture, its norms, rules, prohibitions, rewards, and punishments. If fundamental ethical principles have often been criticized as "abstract" and "acontextual," a similar vagueness accompanies the claim that there are cultures that do not recognize individual persons as basic units, but see them as contributory parts of the society as a whole. It is possible to buy into that premise only after seeing a detailed account of the structure and function of the society. Does it have rituals surrounding death? If so, it recognizes persons as individuals who cease to exist. Does it have rituals surrounding birth? If so, it recognizes persons as individuals who come into being. Does it have sanctions for punishing people who violate the society's rules? If so, it recognizes individuals as moral agents capable of obeying or disobeying the established rules that provide for social order. Does it have a healer, a designated person or persons who minister to sick individuals and seek to heal them (by whatever means)? If so, then the society recognizes human beings as individual persons who deserve care and attention when they fall ill. None of these forms of recognition compels the conclusion that individuals have rights. But we cannot even formulate the questions about birth, death, punishment, or healing without taking the individual person as the unit of analysis. So, the claim that some societies do not recognize individual persons apart from the society of which they are a part is either false or incoherent, at least without a rich description that enables us to make some sense out of the claim.

It is likely, however, that a more accurate statement is the much weaker claim that many societies place the interests of the group above the interests (or rights, if they are recognized) of individual members of the society. That is perfectly consistent with an acceptance of the principles of humanity and humaneness because the two principles are not accorded a fixed order of priority. A society that generally places the interests of the group over the interests of individuals could, on this account, be more morally progressed than a culture in which the individual reigns supreme. But to make that judgment, we would need a full description of the laws, policies, and mechanisms for maintaining social order and providing for social welfare in the societies in question.

Adherents of the postmodern school of thought will not be persuaded by this sort of analysis. That is because postmodernists begin with the denial that there is any objective validity to descriptive statements about cultures or people's roles in them. If everything is socially constructed, there is no underlying reality. If there can be no cultural universals to speak of, there surely cannot be ethical universals. Adherents of the postmodern school of thought reject conclusions drawn from logical arguments because there is no way to confirm the truth of the premises. Postmodernists may also mistrust the rules of logical inference. If all of semantics is socially constructed, the same may be true of syntactics.

For the same reason that it is impossible for an atheist and a religious believer to accept one another's mode of reasoning, it is an exercise in futility to argue with postmodern defenders of ethical relativism. The metaphysical differences in the fundamental premises of the atheist and the religious believer are so vast, there is no starting ground for debate. It is the same with regard to the postmodern denial that there is any objective social reality. If everything cultural is socially constructed, it follows that there can be no ethical universals and no fundamental moral principles applicable to all humankind. My arguments are not directed to postmodern defenders of relativism but to those who, recognizing cultural diversity and the value of tolerance, genuinely wonder how we can talk of human rights and at the same time accept the thesis of ethical relativism. In a deeply challenging dialogue, I tried out the main thesis of this book on a colleague whom I met on an international ethics committee. She is a feminist, a social scientist, and a health advocate, whose work includes both social planning and research. We are both members of a committee at the WHO that reviews the scientific and ethical aspects of research in human reproduction, and our discussion began when I commented on the remarkable agreement this internationally constituted committee manages to achieve at its semiannual meetings in Geneva (current members are from the United Kingdom, Canada, Mexico, Argentina, Thailand, Malaysia, Sweden, Italy, Israel, Bulgaria, Zimbabwe, Japan, and China). The colleague with whom I had the extended dialogue is originally from the Netherlands, currently works in England, and spent 6 years in the bush in Papua New Guinea living in a remote community.

She began with the familiar observation that some cultures do not recognize individuals apart from the community and that in those societies the interests of the community take precedence over those of the individuals. I pressed her for a concrete example, and she provided the following illustration. Western, capitalistic societies recognize the right of individuals to hold property. When one individual's property rights are violated by another person, it constitutes theft or trespass, and the violator can be punished by state-imposed sanctions. In contrast, there are societies that do not recognize individual property rights. All property belongs to the community as a whole and is shared by all. Consequently, in that society, if one individual sought to obtain or maintain a piece of property as a private possession, other members of the society would experience psychological distress and would suffer harm, whereas in the capitalistic society those whose property rights are violated suffer distress and are harmed.

An interesting example. What does it show? First, far from it being the case that the society under discussion does not recognize the individual separate from the community as a whole, the story demonstrates that individuals in that society can suffer psychological harm and the society as a whole acknowledges individual suffering to be harm. My Dutch colleague admitted as much, and refined her point to make the weaker claim that the interests of individuals are subsumed under those of the community as a whole. But then she added: Members of that society could very well argue that having a system of communally shared property is a fundamental value, so it is the capitalistic system of private property that shows less moral progress. Because members of the communal society suffer distress when one of their number seeks to hold private property, more suffering results, on the whole, from a social system that recognizes private property rights than from one that does not.

But it is also true that members of a capitalistic society suffer distress if they are not permitted to hold property, or when their property is confiscated by the government, or when a socialist reform government engages in land redistribution. A system of political economy, such as capitalism or socialism, can be judged by fundamental ethical principles, but the different systems themselves are not inherently just or unjust, morally right or morally wrong. Property rights are not fundamental human rights, they are derivative or intermediate rights. In a capitalistic system, the right to own property is granted to individuals, and in a socialist system the right to a decent minimum standard of living is guaranteed to its members. The right to hold private property is a morally relative value, and it would be an example of cultural imperialism to hold that the nonindustrialized society in which all property is communally held is, for that reason, less morally progressed. Here again, we would need a rich description of the entire social system, its rules, laws, and sanctions, to determine where it stands on a continuum of moral progress. No single feature of a society or culture can be used to ascertain the degree of moral progress of the society as a whole, relative to another culture or society with which it is being compared.

My colleague from the Netherlands agreed that her property rights example could show that some things can legitimately be held to be ethically relative, while others may not be. One aspect of her work in Papua New Guinea was developing interventions to decrease the amount of domestic violence against women and the widespread acceptance of such violence as "normal" and unavoidable. But if the widespread domestic violence in that society (and elsewhere) is simply viewed as an accepted fact of cultural life, attempts at reform could have no moral basis.

Another aspect of her work had been to combat widespread malnutrition, especially of infants, by providing better health education for the mothers. That task included an encouragement to give the babies solid food in addition to breast milk after the first few months of life. Some women objected to providing the additional food, and my friend inquired whether there were reasons apart from the general scarcity of food. One of the mothers said that the ingestion of solid food in a child prior to toilet training would result in foul-smelling feces, and this would be most unpleasant. Despite her defense of ethical relativism, my colleague did not accept that reason as a justification for denying a child nutrients required for health and growth. And when a mother of twins took one of the babies into the forest to leave it to die because the family could not support two infants born at the same time, the Dutch health worker voiced the ethical judgment that infanticide is wrong, although she did not criticize the mother directly when she learned of the episode.

In today's world, we have to analyze ethical relativism by considering two very different types of societies. The first are non-Western societies—countries for the most part in Asia and Africa. Although common parlance continues to distinguish these by calling them *developing* countries, it may be time to change that terminology. The term denotes economic development, a narrow concept that fails to capture the ways in which many of these so-called developing countries in the non-Western world are very much like Europe and North America. One of those ways is the recognition by opinion leaders, academics and professionals, community representatives, and somewhat better-educated citizens, of the existence and importance of human rights. The pronouncements by official spokespersons at United Nations conferences can be a far cry from the views stated at international meetings and workshops where the participants are not governmental officials or political leaders.

The second type of society is radically different from the Western world and from the countries typically referred to as "developing." They exist in many parts of the world, including some parts of Europe as well as North and South America. These societies include tribes, indigenous peoples, remote villages, and other places that have little access to means of global communication and the dialogues, debates, and struggles for human rights. They are the traditional objects of study by anthropologists and are examples of the genuine concept of a distinct culture. Remnants of an isolated world of earlier eras, these remote communities do not explicitly reject the moral values of the West. It is more than likely they are unaware that any such values exist.

To contend that they exhibit a lower degree of moral progress than societies whose laws, policies, and moral discourse adhere to the principles of humaneness and humanity is not to subject them to blame. That is because they are in a state of "culturally induced moral ignorance."[15] As Allen Buchanan writes: "This ignorance exists when enculturated beliefs and concepts prevent individuals from discerning what they ought to do and is nonculpable when individuals cannot be blamed for not escaping the effects of such ignorance."[16] To judge that one society or cultural group is less morally progressed than another does not automatically condemn the former for its failure to live up to the moral standards of the latter. If an entire society can appropriately be characterized in terms of "culturally induced moral ignorance," then the judgment of its lower stage of moral progress is not a condemnation but a descriptive statement.

Culturally induced ignorance may stem from a lack of morally relevant factual information or from a more deep-seated moral ignorance. An example of the former is the Iu Mien mother whose beliefs about medical causes and remedies is so far removed from modern medical science that she has no possible way of determining that she is harming rather than benefiting her child. An example of the latter is the Oriya Brahmans who believe that beating a wife who goes to the movies without her husband's permission is morally justified by the relationship between husbands and wives in the institution of marriage. In relevant respects marriage is like the hierarchical structure in the military. With regard to both types of culturally induced ignorance, inhabitants of such societies are not subject to moral blame but rather are in need of scientific or moral education.

In contrast, members of the first type of society or culture, one that is well acquainted with principles that dictate respect for persons and humane treatment of patients, research subjects, prisoners, captives, and others, cannot offer the excuse that they have been so far removed from the principles, policies, and practices of democracy that they have never heard of human rights. What is most instructive is the difference between the pronouncements of political leaders and rulers in such societies and the views of people who work for the betterment of their fellow inhabitants in the same places. Political leaders in China may well argue that "reproductive rights" is an idea of Western democracies that does not apply to them. The Pope may argue that "reproductive rights" is a goal of radical Western feminists that does not apply to women in poor, developing countries. Religious leaders among Muslims, possibly ignorant of their own religion's teachings, claim that female genital mutilation is required by their religion and therefore should be immune from an ethical critique by the non-Muslim world. None of these groups or spokespersons lacks familiarity with the cultural and ethical perspectives of democratic ideals, respect for the autonomy and the rights of individuals, and other values typically denominated as "Western." Official spokespersons from these cultures simply deny that "Western" values apply to their country, a claim that typically serves their own interest in maintaining the status quo.

What do the people in these countries think? There is a disconnect between the statements of traditional leaders and the views of activists for social reform, academics and professionals, and community leaders who know and care about individual rights, participatory institutions, and other so-called "Western" values. There is a disconnect between the statements of those who defend a status quo perpetuating an oppressive and hierarchical social system, and people from thes same cultures who advocate social change based on ethical principles very much like the principles of humanity and humaneness. Can the beliefs and values of this latter group be explained only under the hypothesis that they are dupes of Western cultural imperialism? That supposition demeans advocates of reform by implying that they are not or cannot be independent thinkers, but are slavish adherents of the Western moral concepts with which they have come into contact and seek to emulate.

To get beyond relativism is not to embrace ethical imperialism. To acknowledge the existence of universal ethical principles is not a commitment to moral absolutism. Ethical principles always require interpretation when they are applied to particular social institutions, such as a health care system or the practice of medicine. In the particulars, there is ample room to tolerate cultural diversity. But our social institutions would still be in the dark ages if we had not progressed to a stage where human rights are recognized and upheld. Once we uphold and promote human rights, we have taken a stance against relativism.

Notes

1. Portions of this chapter are excerpted from my "Moral Progress," *Ethics*, Vol. 87, No. 4 (1077), pp. 370–382.

2. Alison D. Renteln, "Relativism and the Search for Human Rights," *American Anthropologist*, Vol. 90 (1988), p. 57.

3. For a somewhat similar view, see David C. Thomasma, "Bioethics and International Human Rights," *Journal of Law, Medicine & Ethics*, Vol. 25 (1997), pp. 295–306, especially his discussion of Erich Loewy's argument, p. 299.

4. Eric J. Cassell, "Pain and Suffering," (ed.) Warren T. Reich, *Encyclopedia of Philosophy*, 2nd edition (New York: Macmillan, 1995), pp. 1897–1905.

5. Thomasma. pp. 299–303.

6. Thomasma, p. 295.

7. Thomasma, p. 301.

8. Thomasma, p. 301.

9. Burns, pp. 1, 12.

10. Barbara Crossette, "Afghan Women Demanding End to Their Repression by Militants," *New York Times* (April 6, 1998), pp. A1, A8.

11. Elinor Burkett, "God Created Me To Be a Slave," *The New York Times Magazine*, (October 12, 1997), pp. 56–60.

12. Youssef M. Ibrahim, "Algeria to Permit Abortions for Rape Victims," *New York Times* (April 14, 1998), p. A6.

13. Lynn P. Freedman, "Women and the Law in Asia and the Near East," *Genesys*, Special Studies No. 1 (1991), p. 21.

14. Carl Wellman, "The Ethical Implications of Cultural Relativity," (ed.) Paul W. Taylor, *Problems of Moral Philosophy* (Encino, CA: Dickenson Publishing Co., 1972), p. 74.

15. Allen Buchanan, "Judging the Past: The Case of the Human Radiation Experiments," *Hastings Center Report*, Vol. 26, No. 3 (1996), pp. 25–30.

16. Buchanan, p. 27.

Index

multicultural health care team, 130–32
multiculturalism, 110, 113–14, 117–18, 122
organ transplantation and definition of death, 139, 141
privacy, 12
racism, 250
research and ethical imperialism, 188–93, 195–96, 200, 205–06, 210, 214
self-determination, 86
United States Agency for International Development, 203–04
Universal Declaration of Human Rights (1948), 226, 229, 232
Universality
ethical principles, 44–54
reproductive rights, 176–77
research and ethical imperialism, 213
Universals, definition of, 35
University of Delhi, 155
Urbanization, 194
Urinary tract infections, 67
Uruguay, reproductive rights in, 182
Utilitarian moral theories
female genital mutilation, 77
moral progress and ethical universals, 251
philosophers and anthropologists debate, 43–44
reproductive rights, 173

Vaccines, 169–71, 173–75
Validity
cultural and ethical relativism, 19
moral progress and ethical universals, 268
Value accorded to individual person, 9
Value-free stance, anthropological, 68
Value judgements, anthropological, 31, 200
Value neutrality
female genital mutilation, 68, 73, 78–79
reproductive rights, 165
Values
doctor-patient relationship, 100–01
human rights in health and medicine, 227–33
philosophers and anthropologists debate, 42, 49–51
Vatican. *See also Catholic Church*
language of rights, 224

reproductive rights, 175–79, 181
Vesicovaginal fistula, 61–64
Vietnam
human rights, 228
research and ethical imperialism, 206
Village chiefs, research and ethical imperialism, 194–95
"Violence against women," 21–22, 270
Virginity, 78
Virtue-based value systems, 93–94, 104
Visionaries, social, 21
Voluntariness, 76
Voodoo ritual, 115–17
Vulgar relativism, 41–43, 45

Warfare, 194
"Way of life," 6
Wellman, Carl, 262
Western civilization, moral progress and ethical universals, 250
Western culture
bias, 31
confidentiality, 14
death, 263
doctor-patient relationship, 94, 96–98, 104
female genital mutilation, 73–74
imperialism, 54
moral progress and ethical universals, 255
philosophers and anthropologists debate, 32
privacy, 12, 14
Western Europe
doctor-patient relationship, 99
human research subjects, 259
philosophers and anthropologists debate, 30
research and ethical imperialism, 189, 205
Western medicine, 91–92
Western principle of autonomy, 262
"Western rescue missions," 74
"White man's burden," 25
Widows
Hindu, 6, 52, 257–58
research and ethical imperialism, 202–03, 205
Wife beating, 39–41, 242–43, 272
Wife killing, 244